MACULAR DISEASE

Practical Strategies for Living with Vision Loss

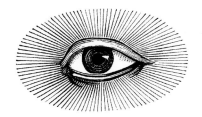

Peggy R. Wolfe

PARK PUBLISHING, INC.
Minneapolis, Minnesota
New Richmond, Wisconsin

First edition

Printed in the United States of America

ISBN-10: 09792945-1-7
ISBN-13: 978-0-9792945-1-8

Library of Congress Cataloging-in-Publication data

Wolfe, Peggy R.
    Macular disease : practical strategies for living with vision loss / Peggy R. Wolfe.
        p. cm.
    Includes index.
    ISBN 978-0-9792945-1-8
    1. Retinal degeneration—Popular works. I. Title.
    RE661.D3W65 2008
    617.7'35—dc22

                                                          2008007781

Editor and publishing consultant: Linda Gray
Cover and interior designer: Monica Baziuk
Indexer: Robert J. Richardson
Proofreader: Maggie Gallivan

Product photographs and trademarks are used in this book for informational purposes only. This book is not endorsed or sponsored by, or otherwise affiliated with, any of the manufacturers or trademark owners.

PARK PUBLISHING, INC.
511 Wisconsin Drive
New Richmond, Wisconsin 54017

9 8 7 6 5 4 3 2 1

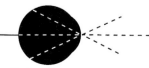

**This Large Print Book carries the
Seal of Approval of N.A.V.H.**

Contents

PART 3
Arranging Your Affairs and Using Assistive Technology 113

Acknowledgments

LIVING THE LAST eight years with gradually decreasing vision has not been a solo journey. I've received support and inspiration along the way from the many guides listed below. Perhaps the only way to thank them is to let them know that the help they have given me is now being transmitted to a wide audience through this book.

I am deeply grateful to the staff at Vision Loss Resources in Minneapolis—both for giving me invaluable advice about this book and for opening new vistas for me as I came to understand all the services offered at the center. I wish to especially acknowledge Ellen Morrow, MA, for her personal counsel and for testing layout samples with her support groups, whose members I thank for the direction they offered. Thanks also to Kate Grathwol, PhD, Jean Christy, and other staff members. My appreciation also goes to instructors of classes, the fellow students in my skills class, and all the inspiring people I have met at Vision Loss Resources.

My earnest thanks to the many medical professionals who provided both excellent care over the years and invaluable support as I wrote this book. I am particularly indebted to my ophthalmologist, Dorothy Horns, MD, for her early detection of my macular degeneration; my retinologist, Robert C. Ramsey, MD, for patiently answering my endless questions at visits during the last eight years, for enrolling me in a research study, for giving advice about the scope of the book, and for his successful treatments as my disease has progressed; and clinical research coordinator Julianne Enloe, CCRP, COA, for her encouragement during the years I was a study participant. Thanks also to my primary care physician, Louise G. Wright, MD, for her early diagnosis of my celiac disease, thus returning me to good health; to my audiologist, Julie A. Klosterman, MS CCC-A, who has guided me in my selection of hearing aids and who offered valuable ideas presented in the section on hearing loss, and to my Pilates instructor, Angela Kneale, OTR, Certified Pilates Instructor, who has helped me develop strength and balance in body and mind and who contributed to the exercise section of this book.

For their advice on low vision and assistive technology products, sincere thanks to Steve Zent at Freedom of Speech and Kevin Nicholson BA, MS, COMT, at Minnesota Low Vision Store.

I would not have been able to write this book without the kindness and support of my friends. Thanks to Arlys

Gribovsky for her feedback on the cover design; Diane Follmer for reading early drafts and offering suggestions on content and layout; Nancy Quinlan, who taught me what it is like to live with diabetic retinopathy and who tested the lamp with magnifier shown in the book; Reiko Ito Shellum-Koeck and Eugene Koeck, my ballet instructors, who have offered both support and patience as I persevere in my balletic attempts; Amy Krane for her generosity in driving me to ballet class; "Taxi Al" Perlman for his good humor and advance scheduling of my taxi rides; Jeanette DesMarais, whose biweekly visits have kept my household in order even while she resisted the temptation to clean up all the piles of papers on my desk and floor; and Mary Salisbury, my inspiring volunteer buddy, who has modeled how to live with personal adversity.

My heartfelt gratitude goes to my family for their support from the moment I had the idea of writing this book. Thanks to my son, Steven Wolfe, for his photographs in chapters 6 and 10 and for taking practice shots for the other photos, as well as for assuming management responsibilities in our publishing business to free my time for writing this book; to my daughter, Katie Wolfe, for being my planning buddy who kept me on track in writing this book, read early drafts, and made sure I had some fun along the way; and to my sister, Jean Richter, for reading and offering suggestions on endless drafts and especially for her emotional support when I was discouraged. To my late husband, Fancher E. Wolfe, my most poignant thanks for his continuing support of my writing this book, even as his health declined.

Finally, but not least, I want to express my deep indebtedness to the people on my team who, through their advice and special talents, have helped bring this book to a high professional level. My enthusiastic appreciation goes to my editor, Linda Gray, for helping me develop and express my thoughts, for her suggestions and corrections, which were always offered with tact and good humor, and for her ardent fact checking; to Monica Baziuk, cover and interior designer, for her astute aesthetic sense and creativity, along with her profound patience and perseverance in developing sample after sample; to Scott Knutson, for his expert photography; to Robert J. Richardson, for his excellent indexing, to Maggie Gallivan, for her precision in proofreading the book; and to Mary Rowles at Independent Publishers Group, for her invaluable advice on the book's concept, her winning title suggestion, and her guidance on selecting the right editor for this project.

Preface

THIS BOOK is being written in real time as I continue to adjust to the progressive decline of my vision from macular degeneration. My goal is to give useful hints to my fellow travelers on the path to living with peripheral vision. Eight years ago, at the age of 69, I was referred by my ophthalmologist to a retinologist, and the diagnosis of early macular degeneration was confirmed. I wasn't too surprised, as my mother and my uncle lived with macular disease for many years. They provided me gutsy examples of how to live with vision loss. This longtime exposure to their stalwart optimism left me with an accepting spirit—one not filled with fear, but with the will to do battle. I've fought back by developing many strategies to make my life easier now and to prepare for the day when I must rely solely on my peripheral vision.

When I was first diagnosed, my retinologist told me about a research study that was testing low-level laser surgery as a way to slow the progress of the disease. When he asked if I'd like to join the study, I immediately agreed. I knew that, even if it didn't help me, it could help others. I was the third patient in the practice to sign on.

The results of multiple studies of this low-level laser treatment showed no statistical advantage over not receiving any treatment. However, another study carried out at about the same time showed that taking a particular vitamin-antioxidant combination slowed the progress of the disease in some cases. At the time of this writing, taking these pills is the best thing we can do to help slow the progression of macular degeneration, and I've done so faithfully.

But when I recently bit the bullet and asked my retinologist how long he predicted I'd be able to read, he guessed one to two years. Rather then discouraging me, this news energized me to increase my pace of preparation and to share what I've learned with others who are in the same situation.

Although I am not a medical professional, I am well informed about the disease. My working life has been spent as a research librarian at a major university, so I'm drawn to research when confronted with a new challenge. I'm also the owner of a small family publishing business, so it seems perfectly natural to me to write a book about the things that have been helpful to me as my sight diminishes. I hope you will find the ideas presented in this book useful.

Peggy R. Wolfe

Introduction

IF YOU ARE living with macular disease, you will benefit from learning about strategies and useful aids that can help you deal with various areas and phases of your life as your vision slowly diminishes. This book provides that information and more.

As a lay person whose expertise comes from having lived with vision loss from macular degeneration for eight years, I do not attempt to include coverage of the medical aspects of macular disease. Rather, the book is a personal guide to dealing with the very real situations and challenges that you have been or may be presented with. It is my goal to offer you real hope, confidence, and optimism about your life with vision loss.

You will find that, although you may need to do things in a different manner, you can still do them. All of us with vision loss experience both fiascos and triumphs, and many of mine are illustrated here in the form of personal stories about some of the experiences I have had as I've learned, and continue to learn, to live with macular degeneration.

About This Book's Design

This large print book was specifically designed for the reader who has limited vision. The goal was to find type that would be easy to read and a layout that would clearly identify the topics. After testing with low vision readers, the results are presented in this volume. It is printed on glare resistant, heavy paper that makes the pages easy to turn. The off-white color provides good contrast against the large, heavy, black type. I hope that you will enjoy handling and reading this book.

How to Use This Book

You may want to skim through the book to get an idea of what is covered, then read those sections that seem most relevant to your life right now. Or you may prefer to read it from cover to cover. I suggest you keep this book in an easy-to-find spot so that you can refer to it whenever a new situation comes up. As you face a new challenge, look in the index for topics that will help you deal with the new problem.

The book has a take-charge approach that offers a positive way of looking at your life now and later. Because macular diseases generally proceed very slowly, my intention is that this book will be your handy companion for many years.

PART 1

Sustaining the Spirit, Mind, and Body

YOU CAN USE your mind and your spirit to find ways to enjoy your life now and to prepare for the future. The first chapter in this section suggests ways to develop this positive approach. The author's own experience is given in the "My Story" features that you will find throughout the book. In chapters 2, 3, and 4 you will find information on how to maximize your vision by using special lighting, caring for your body through diet and exercise, optimizing hearing if you have a loss, and developing your sense of touch and other senses.

Nourishing the Spirit and the Mind

YOUR LIFE, after receiving a diagnosis of a macular disease, may be taking a different course from the one you had been expecting, but it is not a hopeless picture. You will find that you can still do the things you have been doing—but that you will need to do them in different ways. You may feel powerless, but be active in finding solutions to the particular difficulties you may face. Think of yourself as a fighter who will meet the challenges posed by your vision loss, rather than as a victim. Let finding tactics to deal with your disease become your strategic game plan. Become a creative problem solver and use ideas in this book that have worked for others to find solutions that work for you.

Develop a Positive Outlook and Control What You Can

Many things in life have always been beyond our control, from the forces of nature to the behavior of other people. Being confronted with some new limitations in your life does not mean you are suddenly more powerless. There are still many areas of your life that you can control. Change the things you can. Most important of these things is your own attitude. If you are discouraged, develop a determination to rule your own life. As diseases affecting the macula usually have a slow progression, you may have years of declining, but still quite functional, vision. Consider your diagnosis an advance notice—a gift of time to gradually prepare for the day when you may be relying on your peripheral vision. Use this book as a guide to the things you can do in various areas of your life to maintain the independence that will give you confidence and a sense of power.

Be Good to Yourself and Do What Is Most Important to You

You have received a very distressing diagnosis, and you probably feel confused, frightened, and depressed. I suggest that the first thing you do is figure out what the most important things in your life are—the things that bring you the most contentment and joy. Then immediately plan to do one of these things as a special treat to yourself. It should be something that fills your heart with joy. Practical activities required for daily living don't qualify. What you pick need not involve a financial expenditure, but rather the investment and the reward of love and time well spent. Perhaps you'd like to take a walk with a special friend in a beautiful park or visit someone you haven't seen in a long time. Maybe your treat will be enjoying a local museum or going to a concert with a friend. You can save most of your ideas for later times, but this first one should be something really special. Then remember to find ways to be good to yourself on a continuing basis.

——— MY STORY ———

Dream Trip with My Daughter

When my retinologist told me he guessed I had one to two years before I lost my central vision and would no longer be able to read or view objects, I sat down and thought about how this new situation would fit into my life. I decided the first step was to figure out what was most important to me. The answer was twofold—first, to spend time with my daughter, who lives in another state; and second, to experience the great joys of my life—classical music, opera, ballet, and visual arts. This all added up to a trip with my daughter to New York City. It was a special time together, and we visited art museums and attended opera and ballet performances. We shared all expenses, which helped to make the trip possible, and I will always have the memory of our time together, doing things we both love.

Have Some Fun

This idea fits in with finding and doing things that are important to you, but the emphasis here is on relaxing and just enjoying what you are doing. Go to some movies and organize outings with family and friends. If you want to meet people, you can find many activities at senior centers. Most centers have newsletters with monthly calendars of events. You can get games for people with diminished vision and playing cards with large, bold numbers. Maybe your idea of fun and relaxation is simply a slower pace to your life so that you can savor each day.

Allow Yourself to Grieve Your Losses While Moving On to Acceptance

Even as you focus on finding joy in life, understand that you are suffering not only the loss of vision, but also the loss of what you thought the rest of your life would be like. As with any other grief, you may feel shock or disbelief, or even find yourself in denial that this is happening to you. Anger, fear, and questions of "Why me?" are other common reactions. You may experience a profound sadness and have trouble dealing with your anxiety about the future. These are normal and very understandable emotions, and allowing yourself to feel them can help you to accept what has happened and then let go of your fears. If your vision loss—which perhaps comes on top of other losses—causes you significant depression, it may help you, as it has helped others, to seek counseling or a vision loss support group. Be patient and gentle with yourself as you strive for acceptance—it will bring you both peace and the will to move forward to your new "normal" life.

Strengthen Your Spirit by Developing Your Inner Resources

People think of "spirit" in many different ways. One definition is "life force." Helpful qualities that are found within that concept include: backbone, boldness, character, dauntlessness, energy, enterprise, enthusiasm, grit, guts, heart, humor, morale, motivation, resolve, soul, vitality, warmth, and will. Developing these qualities will help you to live a rewarding life with courage and purpose.

Find a Spiritual Home

For many people, belonging to a faith community brings spiritual fulfillment and peace. Membership in churches, synagogues, or other places of worship can lead you to fellowship with people who will give you their comfort and support. If you have not already found such a spiritual home but feel a yearning, this is a good time to start that search.

Nurture Your Mind

Keep your mind active by reading while you are able to do so. You can get books and magazines in large print versions as reading becomes more difficult. If you listen to the radio or TV with your eyes closed, you can develop your listening skills. Get used to listening to books on tape or compact discs or as downloads from the Internet—this skill will come in very handy, as you can become eligible to participate in the free Talking Book Program, a service of the Library of Congress, which is described on pages 136–143. Learn something new by taking classes offered by community education organizations. Most offer courses that teach you how to use a computer, and it would be good to learn how to access the Internet and use e-mail. For one-on-one instruction, ask your children, grandchildren, or friends to teach you. One of them may have an old computer system that he or she will be happy to give you. Developing computer skills will open untold doors for you, and technological advances in accessibility are making computers easier and easier to use.

Volunteer for Rich Rewards

Perhaps the best thing you can do for yourself, while helping others at the same time, is to become a volunteer. You may think you have nothing to offer, but there is an opportunity waiting for you somewhere. Churches, the

United Way, and senior centers are three good places to find the right volunteer work for you. These organizations need volunteers for all types of jobs, so think about your skills and what you enjoy doing, and make a call. If there is a vision rehabilitation center in your community, you can join an advocacy group or work with a staff member in a support group. The possibilities are endless.

MY STORY
First a New Church, Then a Perfect Volunteer Job

I had halfheartedly been looking for a spiritual home over a period of years. I'd attend one church for a few months, then another. I did not feel at home in any of them. Then one Sunday I attended services at a church that I'd been hearing had beautiful music. I had not gone there before because I thought it was too huge a congregation, but as soon as I felt the friendly atmosphere and heard the soloist and choir, I knew this was where I belonged. My search was over and I joined the church right away. Soon I wanted to be more closely involved in its community, so I started looking for a volunteer job among the many offerings. One day the coordinator called, said there was an opening in the music library, and asked if I'd be interested, considering I had a library degree. I said yes, and was soon working with a special woman who has become my "volunteer buddy." Our project is to list in a database each track of every compact disc held in the music library. Our trio of coordinator and two volunteer buddies has developed a close and loving relationship that is very important to each of us. My friendship with these two women has enriched my life beyond words, and the bonus is that I'm working with music, too. These have been great gifts to me.

Gifts that will be important to you are:

- Acceptance
- Patience
- Organization
- Independence
- The realization that life is change
- A fighting spirit

Caring for Your Eyes and Vision

MONITOR YOUR VISION regularly and if you notice changes, see your doctor right away. Take good care of your eyes to keep seeing at the highest possible level.

Do Home Vision Tests If You Have Macular Degeneration

Annual checkups are not enough if you have macular degeneration because you are responsible for monitoring your sight on a regular basis. You can do simple tests at home. Your eye doctor has probably given you an Amsler grid to use to check your own eyes, and you should do this periodically, as directed by your doctor. Make the grid test a habit, and do it in the same location, with the same lighting and at about the same time of day, so you will be able to accurately compare your results with those of your previous tests. Be very aware of what you see with each eye so that you will be able to tell if something has changed since your previous test. Do the test as often as your doctor has directed, but don't become obsessed with the grid, as worry does not promote a positive attitude. Look upon the Amsler grid test as just another of your activities. But if you do notice a change, call for an immediate appointment with your doctor.

There are other important ways to monitor your sight. Develop your own benchmark system to check your vision in each eye. For example, you can test your vision by looking, with each eye, at a bedside clock, your watch, or the bathroom scale, or by reading with each eye to see if the lines are wavy. Choose something that you read every day or at least every week, such as a TV listings guide, a newspaper, or a program for religious services. Also, take note if you suddenly need more light for a particular task or if you develop a new sensitivity to glare. Take a proactive approach to monitoring your vision, and take fast action if you notice a change that could require immediate treatment.

Contact Your Doctor If You Notice a Change in Your Vision

Regardless of your particular disease, make an appointment to see your doctor right away if you notice a change in your vision. Although there are no treatments for the dry type of macular degeneration at the time of this writing, there are treatments for the wet type, and research is being conducted on possible future treatments of both the dry and wet forms. Treatments are also available for other diseases that can affect the macula.

If you notice a change in either eye:

- Act immediately, in time for helpful treatment.
- If you have trouble getting an immediate appointment, be an advocate for yourself and keep insisting that you see the doctor.
- Do not procrastinate!

Visit Your Eye Doctors Regularly for Checkups and Tests

It is very important to have complete eye examinations every year. When dealing with macular disease, it is best to see a retinologist who specializes in retinal and macular diseases. You should also see an ophthalmologist on an annual basis for a general eye checkup and for a possible adjustment to the prescription for your eyeglasses.

Keep a copy of your eyeglass prescriptions in your wallet, along with the phone numbers of both your ophthalmologist and retinologist, in case you lose or break your glasses when you are out of town. If you have a sudden change in vision when you are away, be prepared to call your retinologist for advice and a possible referral to a doctor in the area you are visiting. For a longer stay away from home, it would be a good idea to go prepared with the name and contact information of a retinologist that your doctor recommends. The new doctor will call your home retinologist to get your history, including treatments you have received.

At retinology appointments the doctor will check your distance vision by having you read rows of letters on a distant chart. Then you will probably be asked to read from a small card that has rows of either text or numbers in decreasing sizes of type. This card tests the near vision that you use for reading and other close work. If you have macular degeneration, you may be asked to check your eyes with an Amsler grid, as you are doing at home. These vision tests will probably be followed by a glaucoma test. Then you will be given drops to dilate your pupils so the doctor can see into the back of your eyes.

Depending on your diagnosis, further tests may be conducted. Two types of photographs may be taken with a special camera. One type involves color photography. The other is a fluorescein angiography. For these photos, a special dye is injected into a vein in your hand or arm. As the dye circulates through the bloodstream and eventually reaches the eye, the blood vessels in the retina are made visible to the special camera, which takes flash photographs of the eye every few seconds for several minutes. These photo sessions can be difficult to endure because very bright light is flashed into your eyes, but the photos help the doctor determine changes or abnormal blood vessels. The fine detail shown in the photos, when enlarged, make the fluorescein angiography an accurate and valuable tool that is used in the diagnosis of many eye conditions.

Another test, called ocular coherence tomography (OCT) but informally called a scan, obtains high-resolution cross-sectional images of the retina. It is used in the diagnosis of a host of macular diseases. It is also used to follow up on responses to various types of treatment. For example, if you have macular degeneration and bleeding is suspected or if you have had injections in your eye, you will probably have OCT scans at each visit. The scans are less uncomfortable than the photos because there are no bright flashes of light and the duration of the test is shorter.

Shortly after the tests, the doctor will look at the results and explain them to you. Try to have someone present with you, as it helps to have another pair of ears to be sure you do not miss something important when you may be flustered and nervous. It is a good idea to come prepared with a written list of questions and to take notes of the doctor's responses to your questions. Also, have your companion write down the information the doctor gives about the results of your test, possible treatments, and suggestions for your home care. Some people bring a tape recorder so they can listen to everything again later. At my own visits, a number of different people have each come as my support person—my husband, son, daughter, and a cousin from Ireland who was in the country and who also had an appointment. These visits are a good way to help your family members understand your disease and how it is progressing.

Bleeding in the Right Eye—and Then the Left?

I used to think that the telltale sign of bleeding in the eye would be some wild vision distortion such as seeing a clock face as twisted, or print in a book or newspaper as a blur of crooked lines. But my retinologist always ended each visit by asking that I call if I noticed even a small change in either eye.

On my 77th birthday I was feeling very confident because I'd passed the vision test for renewing my driver's license two weeks earlier, much to my surprise. Yet I was trying not to admit to myself that something had changed in my right, "good," eye. That Sunday at church, where I gratefully use the large print program, for the first time I'd found that I could not read the ends of lines or see the music to sing. At home, glare from my computer screen had become intense. I had to change to different types of light bulbs in the dining room, where I have my morning coffee while I read the newspaper—which had suddenly become quite blurry with wavy lines. I was able to pinpoint the problem to my right eye because I was in the habit of testing my vision by reading the daily paper first with one eye, then the other. I usually did vision checks throughout each day, too, by looking at stationary distant objects.

I did not want to make the call to the doctor because I was afraid, but my son's words about the importance of caring for my vision kept ringing in my ears, and I made the call after a few days. My retinologist looked at my dilated right eye and said he saw bleeding, the sign that my dry macular degeneration had turned into the wet kind. To confirm the diagnosis, he ordered a fluorescein angiogram with the dye and an OTC scan. The diagnosis was confirmed. The doctor said he was very surprised, because I was young to have developed the wet form of macular degeneration. He said he was amazed that I'd noticed the change because the bleeding was so slight, and he bemoaned the people who don't notice changes or put off seeing a doctor for six months—at which point, treatment is less able to help.

Before I left the office, treatment was started. I received an injection of Avastin in my right eye that we hoped would halt the bleeding so that my sight would stay at its present level. Almost immediately my vision actually improved, and when I went for my six-week checkup and another injection, we found that my vision had improved to the point that it had been before the bleeding. At the twelve-week point, my vision had continued to improve, but I had another injection as planned. Now, at the six-month point since my first injection, my right eye vision has remained stable and I have had no further injections. I continue to have OTC scans to check for bleeding every six weeks.

Shortly after the second injection, I noticed a change in my left eye when using the Amsler grid. This time I called the doctor's office immediately, and I got an appointment that same day. My retinologist saw no bleeding, and a fluorescein angiogram and OTC scan confirmed that the problem was further degeneration of cells in the macula.

Special Eye Vitamins for Macular Degeneration

Follow your doctor's recommendations about taking the vitamin supplement known as the AREDS formula. It is available over the counter in various versions. In addition to the original hard, orange tablets that are taken in doses of two in the morning and two in the evening, there are soft gelcaps. At first glance, the gelcaps may seem to cost more than the original tablets, but the dosage is only one in the morning and one in the evening, so the gelcaps end up costing less than the tablets.

Both the AREDS formula tablets and gelcaps contain beta-carotene (vitamin A), but not lutein (another naturally occurring carotenoid that aids in eyesight). Some manufacturers make a version of the AREDS formula that contains lutein, but not beta-carotene. This particular version can be difficult to identify because the supplement may not feature AREDS in its name. You may hear this type referred to as "smoker's AREDS," so called because smokers (and sometimes former smokers) are advised to avoid beta-carotene supplements.

Protect Your Eyes from the Sun

It is generally recommended that you protect your eyes from the sun when you are outdoors. If you are affected by glare, such protection is necessary for your comfort. Glare is also a problem for some people when they are in a car and even when they are indoors. Wide-brimmed and visor hats and sunglasses can provide protection. The best type of sunglasses is also among the least expensive.

These NoIR wraparound, fit-over sunglasses offer 100 percent ultraviolet protection. They also help prevent glare and block blue light. The model shown here is excellent

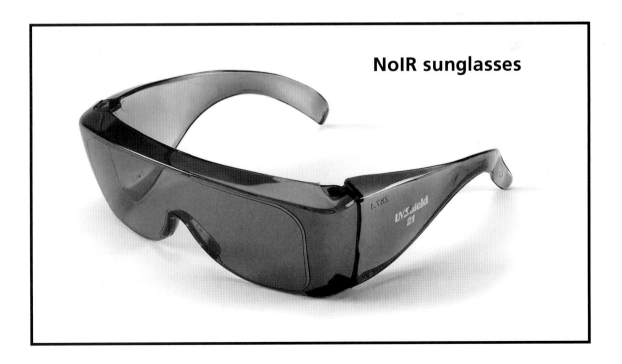

NoIR sunglasses

because it prevents sun from coming in from the sides. The sunglasses are very reasonably priced. They come in various sizes and lens colors—the color you should select depends on your eye condition, as different colors are recommended for diabetic retinopathy, macular degeneration, and retinitis pigmentosa. You can visit the NoIR Web site to see photos of the various colors available. A large selection of NoIR sunglasses is available through the low vision stores listed in Appendix A, and some of these stores' catalogs have helpful charts showing suitable sunglasses colors for various eye diseases.

Increase Your Field of Vision

You may be able to see a wider area at one time by doing relatively simple things like getting glasses for both near and far distances and keeping smudges off you glasses, or by undergoing the more complicated procedure of surgery to fix drooping eyelids, which can cover up to half of the eye in some cases.

Get Both Reading and Distance Glasses— and Keep Them Clean

Having the proper glasses for both near-sight activities, such as reading, writing checks, and sewing, and far-sight activities, such as driving and watching television, allows you to have maximum field of vision at both far and close distances. If you currently wear bifocal or trifocal glasses, you might benefit from getting separate reading and distance glasses so that you will have larger visual fields for both close work and distance work.

A smudge on your glasses can cause a big scare. Often when I start to read it seems that my vision has suddenly gone. But when I hold my glasses up to the light, I see smudges and specks. I wear my reading glasses on a chain around my neck, and the way the lenses hang down seem to make them a magnet for specks and dust. I immediately clean the lenses, and all is well. Place handy bottles of glasses cleaner in every room so it will be easy to clean your glasses, and get tall bottles so you'll be able to spot them.

Fix Drooping Eyebrows and Eyelids with Surgery Covered by Medicare

As one grows older, the upper eyelids can sometimes droop and block the upper field of vision. This can give the appearance of half-open eyes. One cause of drooping is reduced tone in the muscles that control the eyelids. This condition can also be caused by eyebrows that droop so much they make the eyelids droop as well. If your vision is impaired because this drooping limits your field of vision, Medicare should cover approved surgical procedures to correct the problem. A direct brow lift fixes drooping eyebrows, and it is a fairly simple procedure. It is not the same as a forehead lift—a procedure that is done for cosmetic purposes, is very expensive, and is not covered by Medicare.

If it is your eyelids themselves that are drooping, understand that the surgery required to correct the problem is much more complicated. Talk to your doctor and consider your options carefully before proceeding.

─────────── **MY STORY** ───────────

Seeing Better and Looking Younger

Several years ago my visual field became severely obstructed by drooping eyelids, and my doctor sent me to an ophthalmic plastic surgeon for evaluation. His diagnosis was that my eyebrows were drooping so much that they made my eyelids droop also. He took digital photos and sent them to my health insurer to see if my condition met the guidelines for Medicare coverage in my state. The answer was yes, and I had a simple procedure called a "direct brow lift," in which excess skin from my forehead was removed in a wrinkle above my eyebrows. I went to a cookout the next day, wearing sunglasses that covered my eyebrows. No one was the wiser. Prior to my surgery the doctor had taken "before" photos, and, after a few weeks, the "after" photos were taken. The difference was startling, and the wrinkles above my eyebrows looked no worse than they had before the surgery. There were tiny scars but, as they were right in the wrinkles, they were barely noticeable, and they faded away with time. I've retained my "younger," wide-eyed look all these years, and having a full field of vision has been helpful as my sight declines.

Improving Reading Ability

A WELCOME SURPRISE may be in store for you if you think you can no longer read or are finding reading to be an increasingly difficult and frustrating experience. Sometimes all that is needed is properly placed, adequate lighting. Proper lighting provides the contrast that is required to distinguish the letters in words and to distinguish the type from the paper on which it is printed. Newspapers are especially difficult to read, as they are printed on dull, grayish paper, with little contrast between the type and the paper. With macular degeneration, the light-sensing cells in the macula weaken and begin to break down as the disease progresses. This means that a greater amount of external light is needed to read. With diabetic retinopathy and macular degeneration, properly placed light is especially important, as these diseases can cause a great sensitivity to glare. By positioning lamps so that the light is coming from above or behind you, you will help prevent glare.

Reading Stands

Experiment to find the best angle and height to view reading material—sometimes holding it upright and perhaps tilting it back, rather than laying it flat on a table, makes reading much easier.

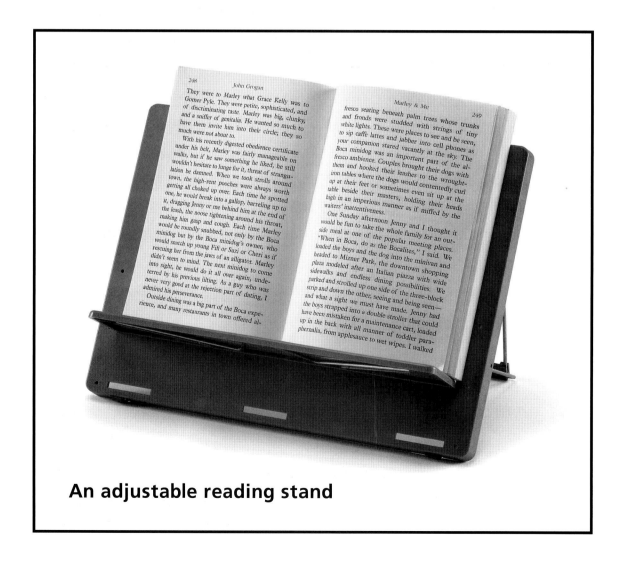

An adjustable reading stand

You can also make reading easier by using a reading stand. A reading stand is a handy way to maintain the best position of your reading material. If you usually need to move your material to the left or right to match a "good spot" in your eye, you may find a reading stand helpful, as it allows you to move or tilt your head while keeping the reading material stationary. This may be easier for you than moving your book or papers around.

The stand in the photo, for example, can be set at four different angles and at three different heights. It holds all types of reading material, from a small book to an oversized atlas to a five-inch-wide, triple-thick three-ring binder. It is especially good for propping up a newspaper to read. The use of a stand also reduces arm and neck fatigue and promotes erect posture, encouraging the proper body alignment that is required for good balance. There are many other styles of reading stands, sometimes called copy holders, book holders, or book stands. Check office supply and low vision stores.

Magnifying Glasses With and Without Lights

Sometimes magnification will enlarge print enough so that you are able to read it. Magnifying glasses are available at several magnification levels, from the lowest level, 2x, up to 15x in a few models. Try different magnification levels, starting with the lowest, until you find the one that works for you now. Do not "buy ahead" in case you need stronger magnification later on. Get the correct strength for your current vision. Go with the minimum magnification level required, because the higher the level, the smaller the view—you will see fewer letters and words as the magnification increases, even when the dimensions of the magnifiers used remain consistent.

Magnifying glasses come in various shapes, sizes, and styles. One unusual style, called a pendant, features a rectangular or round magnifier that hangs around the neck on a cord or chain, keeping the magnifier always handy.

Magnifying glasses are also available with battery-operated lights that make it easier to read because they illuminate the reading material. This is especially useful in low-light conditions. Low-priced illuminated magnifiers with LED lights come in powers ranging from 2x to 15x.

There are also several types of binoculars that attach to your glasses or to a visor. Sports spectacles have the binoculars attached to a frame. These products are good for watching sporting events, TV, and movies, and for other distance viewing tasks. Consult your low vision catalogs to see all the choices.

If you require greater magnification than that provided by magnifying glasses, you may want to consider getting one of the magnification systems that incorporate advanced technology. These systems are discussed in chapter 9.

Choosing Lamps to Fit the Task

For reading and close work, portable lamps—such as floor lamps, table lamps, and clip-on lights—provide good sources of direct lighting. Several types of lamps are discussed in this chapter. Lamps in ceiling fixtures generally do not provide good light for reading, can produce glare, and can't be aimed where you need the light to go. It is also difficult to change bulbs in ceiling fixtures. For these reasons, lighting from ceiling fixtures is not discussed in this book.

Floor Lamps With and Without Magnifiers

Torchiere lamps provide good general lighting that is easy on the eyes because it is indirect, with the light directed upward by a bulb in a reflecting bowl. Some models have a second, lower lamp on the pole that can give light for reading. Inexpensive models of torchiere lamps are available in chain stores.

A more substantial, and expensive, type of lamp has a magnifying lens attached, either at the light source or on a separate arm. These lamps allow your hands to remain free for reading and performing other tasks. They come in both table and floor models, and various types accommodate incandescent, fluorescent, halogen, and "full spectrum" lightbulbs.

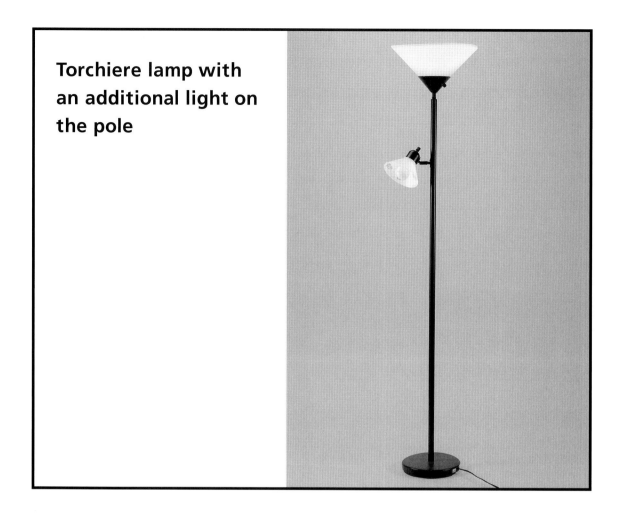

Torchiere lamp with an additional light on the pole

A Giraffe Lamp™ with a rimless magnifier on the end of an adjustable arm is shown in the photo. This lamp has a 30-inch flexible gooseneck and a stationary anti-tip base. The height adjusts from two to seven feet. This is a particularly useful floor lamp because the long neck can easily be twisted to direct the light where you want it. The first item I bought when my vision declined to the point that I wanted better lighting—two and a half years after my diagnosis—was a Giraffe Lamp without the magnifier. I especially like this lamp because I can swing it around to where I want it in a second, then bend it up or down as needed. As an extra bonus, the lamp swivels. Many other brands and models of lamps with magnifiers are also available from low vision stores.

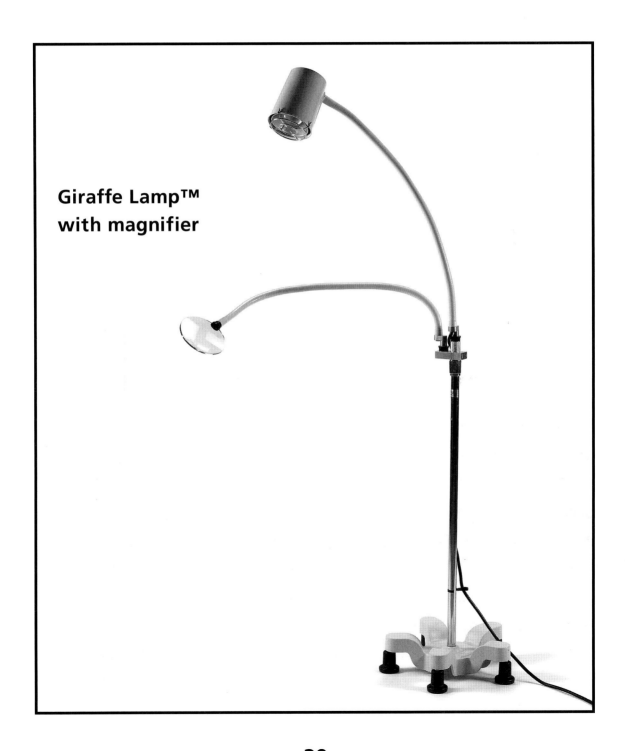

Giraffe Lamp™ with magnifier

Desk and Table Lamps

Traditional table lamps with lampshades do not provide a way to direct light to where you need it to read or perform tasks such as writing checks, balancing checkbooks, or doing craft projects. When you select a lamp for a table or desk, choose one with a flexible gooseneck that can be turned to direct light where it's needed. Small lamps, like the one shown in the next photo, can be found in office supply and discount stores and are reasonably priced. Look for a lamp that comes with a halogen bulb if you want really strong light. Place task lamps to your side to avoid reflected glare from your work surface. Never look directly at a bare bulb that is turned on.

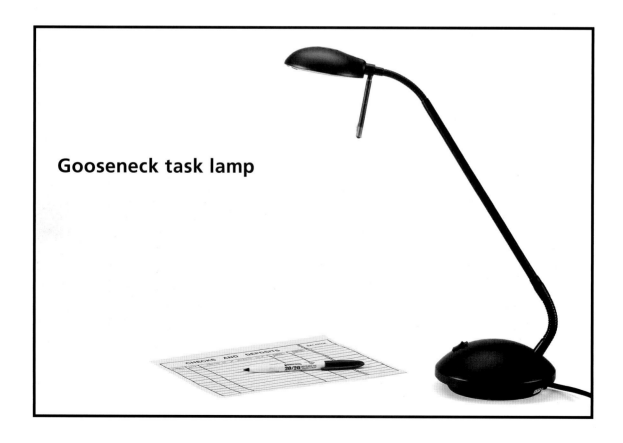

Gooseneck task lamp

If you need more help, you may want to consider a magnifying desk lamp. This type of lamp has a high-intensity bulb and powerful magnification. These lamps cost less than the magnifying floor models.

Clip-on lamps are very useful for attaching a light source to a desk, a computer stand, or the headboard of a bed. These lamps are widely available in discount and home center

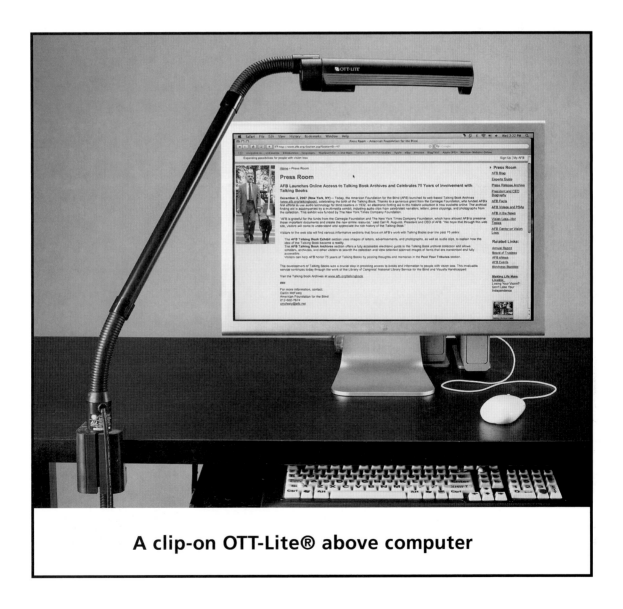

A clip-on OTT-Lite® above computer

stores. The brand shown in the photo on page 31 is an OTT-Lite®, which uses a full-spectrum bulb.

Spot Lighting

When you need to aim light at a particular spot, use a small lamp that directs the light right at the object you want to see. I use a small clip-on lamp above my microwave oven, positioned so that it shines light on the oven's buttons. When I first bought this oven, I could easily read the buttons' white numbers on the black background, but after a couple of years I could no longer detect them—the entire control panel appeared black. The small light allows me to easily see the numbers once again.

Flashlights

Perhaps the most indispensable type of light is the flashlight. One type of small handy flashlight is the pen light. You can use it to direct light at a line of text, such as a line on a menu or in a book. These lights come in models that feature bright LED bulbs. The small flashlights shown in the photo can stand up because they have each been placed in a device called the Flashlite Friend™. This tool also allows the flashlight to remain pointed downward—a useful position for aiming light at a menu or a plate in a dark restaurant. Servers are always fascinated by the way the flashlight can stand in so many positions. The small, six-inch flashlights shown here have also been wrapped in reflective tape to make them easy to spot, even in the dark.

It is a good idea to have several flashlights, each in a Flashlite Friend, available so you can find one when you need it. When placing flashlights around the house, stand them on end, as shown in the center, so they'll be easy to find in the dark—this is especially handy when you need to find a light quickly during a power outage. When you are going out, you can fold the legs of the Flashlite Friend and put the flashlight in your pocket or purse. It is strongly recommended that you keep one in your purse at all times

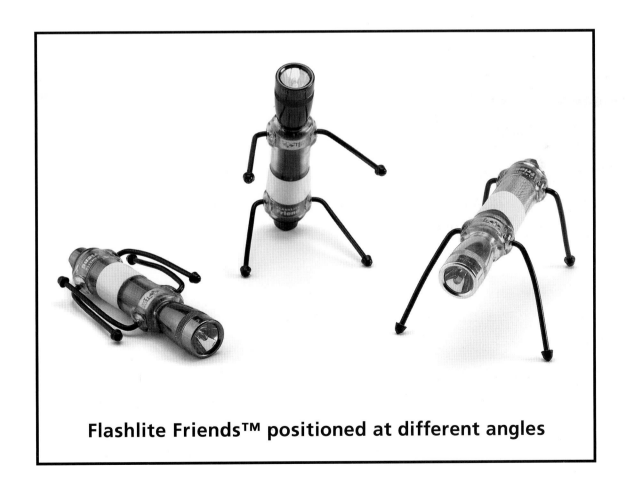

Flashlite Friends™ positioned at different angles

so that you're never accidentally left without one when you're away from home.

Handy Places to Keep Flashlights

In the car—a must

In the kitchen, to help find things in the refrigerator and in cupboards

By your bed, to help you when you get up at night

In your purse or pocket—indispensable at dimly lit restaurants, both for reading the menu and, propped up, for seeing your food

By thermostats, if you need to adjust the settings

By chairs and tables, so that you can find things that fall

On your bureau, to help you see contents of drawers and locate items

Never leave home without a flashlight!

Lantern-Style Flashlights for Power Outages

Lantern-style flashlights provide strong lighting during power outages. Three models are shown here. They each have a handle that makes it easy to carry, but even so, it is a good idea to have two or three lanterns so you can place them in various rooms in the event of a power outage. Find a special place to keep the lanterns when they're not in use so that they are easily accessible. I have three lanterns of different styles, and I keep them on top of the refrigerator because I know I can always find an object that large, even in the dark. I position each of my lanterns with the handle facing outward so I don't have to grapple in the dark to pick one up.

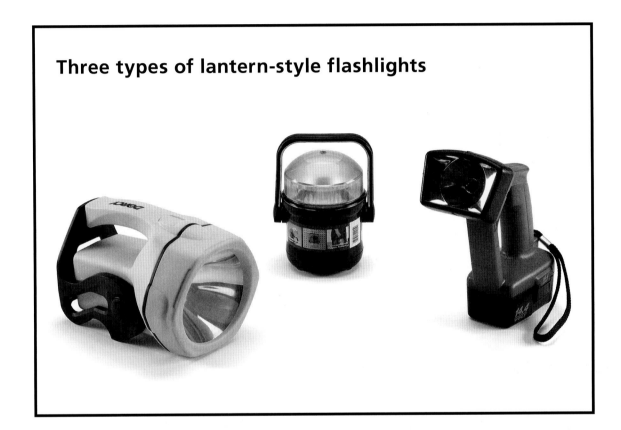

Three types of lantern-style flashlights

Night Lights

Although they are not for reading, night lights are very important for helping you find your way in the dark. They should be in your bedroom, bathroom, hallways, and any other areas where you are likely to walk at night.

Choosing the Best Type of Lightbulb for Your Current Needs

Selecting lightbulbs can be a confusing experience because that are so many types and sizes. The following descriptions should help you select the type that is best for your needs.

- **Incandescent.** This is the type of bulb you grew up with. It is a reliable light source, but it is not energy efficient and it burns out more quickly than newer types, so you have to change the bulbs often.

- **Compact fluorescent.** These bulbs are available in many shapes and sizes that screw into regular, Edison-style sockets. They are more expensive than incandescent bulbs, but they last much longer and more than pay for themselves in energy savings. Using these bulbs, you can save money and conserve energy at the same time. They come in warm, cool, and full-spectrum colors, and they do not have the annoying flutter that long fluorescent tubes sometimes have.

- **Halogen.** This type of bulb is useful for track and task lighting. Halogen bulbs come in a variety of sizes and shapes, with bulbs for track lighting available in angles from 13 to 60 degrees. As my vision has declined, I have moved to the 40-degree bulbs, as the larger angle covers more territory.

■ **Natural daylight or full spectrum.** These bulbs provide light that simulates natural daylight. Many people who are troubled by glare find these bulbs restful. They are available both as incandescent and compact fluorescent bulbs

As your vision changes over time, you will want to experiment with different types of bulbs in your various lamps. In the early stages of your disease you may not even need special lighting, as was my case for more than two years. As time passes you should keep trying different bulbs until you find the best type for each particular lamp and location. Realize that your needs can keep changing, so keep trying until you find the best lamp-bulb combination for you at that particular time. Remember that what works well for you now may not work well for you in the future, so keep experimenting throughout the years to see if a different bulb might allow you to see more clearly.

─────────────── **MY STORY** ───────────────

Glare Led Me to Switch Types of Bulbs

Another symptom of the problem in my right eye was a sudden sensitivity to glare. I could no longer read in the dining room, where I had always read the newspaper. My dining room has two light sources—a Giraffe Lamp and an overhead fixture. Fortunately, I keep a supply of four different kinds of bulbs—incandescent, compact fluorescent, full spectrum, and halogen. When I found the glare in the dining room overpowering, I replaced the halogen bulb in the Giraffe Lamp with a full-spectrum bulb, and the incandescent bulb in the ceiling fixture with a compact fluorescent bulb. Now I am again comfortable reading in that room, and if my needs change I will again try different combinations of bulbs.

4

Nurturing Your Body

YOU HAVE MANY SENSES in addition to sight, and this is the time to start fine-tuning them. In addition to the five commonly known senses of sight, hearing, taste, touch, and smell, there are two others that are especially important to people with vision loss. The first is the perception of balance. The second is the perception of your own body—the awareness of your posture and positioning and feelings of movements of your body. These are senses that people are frequently not aware of, but rely on enormously.

It is important to develop the sensory systems mentioned above because they will become more and more important as time goes on. It is also important to work on improving your general physical well-being and fitness level.

Guidelines for a Healthy Lifestyle for You and Your Family

The eye, like any other part of the body, benefits from a healthful diet. Suggested guidelines for a healthy lifestyle from the National Eye Institute of the U.S. National Institutes of Health and from retinologists are listed below. The recommendations are important for everyone, but they are particularly important for anyone who has a macular disease, as well as for his or her children and grandchildren, as macular diseases frequently have genetic components. In my own case, my mother, uncle, and a first cousin all developed a macular disease, and we've traced it back to both the maternal and paternal sides of my mother's family. It is important for both you and your family to follow these suggestions.

- Exercise and increase physical activity.
- Eat a healthful diet high in fruits, green leafy vegetables (especially kale and spinach for macular degeneration), and fish.
- Watch your weight and reduce your fat intake.
- Maintain normal blood pressure and cholesterol levels.
- Do not smoke.
- If you have diabetes, it is important to control your levels of blood sugar, blood pressure, and blood cholesterol. Doing so will help pervert progression of diabetic retinopathy.

Doctors recommend that your children have annual eye examinations, even if they do not require eyeglasses, starting at age fifty. At the appointment, they should tell the doctor about the family history of macular disease. It is also especially important that they not smoke and that they control their weight and do not allow themselves to become obese.

Develop Your Senses of Balance and Body Awareness by Exercising

Exercise becomes more important as vision decreases. We don't realize how much we rely on looking ahead at objects to anchor ourselves in the space we occupy, so it is important to develop our inner balance and body awareness. During exercise, your brain and your muscles learn to communicate more efficiently. Exercise will help you maintain and build confidence in the way your body moves. Being active helps ensure that you can maintain your independence, including your ability to do daily activities such as walking, shopping, bathing, dressing, and cooking. Motivating yourself to start exercising can be difficult, but physical activity is crucial to nurturing your body. You do not need to excel at sports to gain from and enjoy exercise, and you can start at any age and still receive great benefits.

Exercise for Independence

Before starting an exercise program, make an appointment with your doctor, who may offer suggestions on specific types of exercise from among the types listed on the next page.

- Aerobic exercise to improve cardiovascular fitness, immune function, cognitive function, and mood

- Strength training to build and maintain muscle and bone mass

- Flexibility training to improve motion throughout each of your body's joints

- Balance training to develop confident movement

Although each type of exercise is important, balance training is especially critical for someone with vision loss because of the danger of falling when it is difficult to see.

Follow the suggestions below when developing your general fitness program.

- Consult health professionals, such as physical and occupational therapists, for a determination of your strengths and areas of deficit.

- Add their recommendations for balance training to your exercise program.

- Join a class that includes balance exercises.

- Work to develop a good internal sense of balance and the ability to quickly right yourself when thrown off balance.

- Wear shoes with good fit and support and with soles that prevent slipping, but that don't excessively grip the floor.

- Remember that when you are tired, stressed, or distracted, you may respond poorly to challenges, so take extra care.

- Get adequate rest, because it helps ensure quick responses by body and mind.

- Learn exercises and do them in short periods of five to ten minutes throughout the day—you'll benefit just as much from the combined sessions as you would from one long session.

Find a Class to Start Your Exercise Program

After consulting your doctor, it is a good idea to join a class to stay motivated and to receive instruction on how to properly perform exercises. Classes are offered in community recreation centers, community education programs, senior centers, churches, and low vision organizations. If you belong to a health club, you can get individual instruction from a trainer, who can design a program for you.

You might find it helpful to attend classes in yoga, Pilates, and tai chi. Tai chi is especially helpful because it will help you develop inner balance without relying on focusing on a spot in the distance, which you are probably now using to anchor yourself when doing balance exercises. Choosing physical activities that you enjoy will encourage you to practice consistently at home to gain optimal benefits.

If you are physically unable to take a class or do standing exercises at home, you can do chair exercises sitting right in your own living room. Most states have a service that provides a closed-circuit radio network with special programming for those who are unable to read or hold reading material. An exercise program is often included in the service's scheduled programming. My mother faithfully did her chair exercises even though she had severe arthritis and only peripheral vision. These sessions helped her keep a positive attitude and seemed to make her feel better. You can find a radio station in your area by checking the International Association of Audio Information Services' Web site at http://iaais.org/locateservice.html or by calling your state's department of services for the blind. You can also listen to broadcasts of these radio programs on the Internet. See pages 196–197 for more information on these radio services.

Consider That Strength and Agility Are Needed for Driving

Everyone wants to keep driving as long as possible, but often we believe good vision is all that is required for driving. Stop to think about all the muscle groups you use when you drive, and you will understand how exercise can help keep you behind the wheel.

Just to get into the car you need strong leg and upper body muscles. Once you start to drive, you use foot, ankle, and calf muscles for braking and accelerating. Your arms, wrists, and fingers are needed for steering and using dashboard controls. You must have agility to be a safe driver. Your neck must be flexible and strong to be able to turn to check blind spots when changing lanes. Torso strength and agility are needed so that you can twist to the left and right to see what is behind you when preparing to back up. Ankles must be flexible to push the pedals. Driving is definitely a full-body activity.

See chapter 10 for a more detailed discussion of driving.

----------------- **MY STORY** -----------------

An Athletic Failure, But a Lover of Exercise

As a child, teenager, and college student, I tried one sport after the other, both in school gym class and at neighborhood ball games. No matter whether it was softball, basketball, volleyball, swimming, or, finally, golf— I was the person who was not wanted on any team. I totally lacked whatever it is that makes one able to perform at even a minimum level in sports.

Then, in my early 20s, I discovered an adult beginners' ballet class and found the joy of dance. Although I was not innately talented, I was able to do the classic exercises at the barre, and I advanced to work in the center of the room, where there is nothing to hang onto. I continued classes for a few years, then stopped until my late 40s, when I found another adult beginners' class. My love of balletic exercise was renewed, and I took classes for another couple of years.

Thirty years passed until I found, through a very fortunate connection, a ballet class for mature adults offered through my community's education program. By then I was 74 years old, and my body had forgotten everything it had once known about ballet. But my teachers, a husband-and-wife team, were tolerant, and they welcomed me into both their beginning and intermediate classes.

Through another lucky connection, I discovered Pilates, a mind-body exercise system with an approach to movement that emphasizes body alignment, breathing, strength, flexibility, balance, and endurance. My instructor, who is also an occupational therapist, knew exactly how to help me develop the strength and balance I needed to move forward with my study of ballet.

These exercise activities bring me a feeling of exhilaration, and they have given me a level of fitness that has helped me through some trying times when I was coping with both my own health problems and those of my husband. I need the sustenance of body and spirit that exercise provides.

Develop Your Sense of Touch

Start thinking about your sense of touch, which you may have been taking for granted. It will become more important as your vision decreases because touch can help compensate for diminished sight. You feel through nerve endings that act as touch receptors through your skin. Your fingertips are especially sensitive because they have more receptors than most other parts of the body. Just think about how much a small paper cut on the tip of your finger hurts.

This sensitivity allows you to feel the difference between rough and smooth, soft and hard, hot and cold, and wet and dry. Feeling an object will tell you if it is flat or raised, round or square. Certain objects can give you pleasure just by touching and feeling them. In later chapters you will learn how your sense of touch is important in the kitchen and in finding hard-to-spot things that have been identified with special marks.

Find Pleasure in Feeling Various Textures and Objects

Some items that give sensory pleasure when touched or stroked are fabrics such as fleece or velvet, rocks, smooth or textured glass, and wood or metal objects such as sculptures. Petting your cat or dog gives pleasure to both you and your pet. Hugs are felt through your skin, and they can make you feel good all over and can reduce stress. Start looking for things you enjoy feeling and touching to enjoy now—and later.

Practice Identifying Objects by Their Feel and Shape

As you go about your daily activities, become aware of the shapes and sizes of objects you use throughout the day. When you put away dishes, for instance, you can tell the difference between large and small plates and bowls and short and tall glasses. This will enable you to put things in their designated places in your cupboards even if it's difficult to see where they should go. You can learn to tell the difference between knives, forks, and spoons by their shapes and weights. I remember family celebrations and watching my mother and her brother, my Uncle Matt, put away silverware after the feast. I can hear her now saying, "You can tell the good silverware by its heft and weight. Keep it separate from the everyday knives and forks."

Optimize Your Sense of Hearing

As sight diminishes, hearing becomes more and more important. We may not realize how frequently we use our hearing in many areas of our lives, such as when driving— a strong motivation to have your hearing tested if you suspect a hearing loss. As your sight diminishes, hearing will become more important because you need it to connect with other people and to listen to books and other printed material that have been recorded in audio form.

Get Your Hearing Checked

It is best to have your hearing checked by a licensed audiologist to ensure that you receive a thorough examination. If you go to an ear doctor for an examination, the doctor can probably refer you to an audiologist if you need a hearing aid. Simply responding to an ad you receive in the mail for a "free hearing evaluation" may not result in the comprehensive evaluation you require. Because Medicare covers the costs of hearing tests, the cost of getting your hearing tested by a reputable, licensed audiologist should not be an issue. It is important that you entrust your hearing only to a qualified professional.

Licensed audiologists may work in private practices or in hospitals or clinics. If there are underlying medical issues that are causing your hearing to be affected, your audiologist may refer you to an ENT (Ear, Nose, and Throat) physician. If your hearing tests show that you would be helped by a hearing aid, the audiologist will discuss a variety of hearing aid choices with you.

If you have a hearing loss, you will greatly benefit from getting hearing aids. Unfortunately, they are expensive, and they are not covered by Medicare. Some health insurance plans pay a portion of the cost, but usually not every year—every three years is a common period. If the price is out of your reach, discuss your situation with your audiologist—sometimes arrangements can be made for a manufacturer or other source to help you with the expense.

Changing Hearing Aid Batteries

Use of a hearing aid involves the sense of touch. It requires good finger dexterity to put a hearing aid in your ear. Although removal is easier, it still requires dexterity. It is quite possible to accidentally drop an aid on the floor. A bigger challenge is handling the batteries.

My first two hearing aids were completely-in-the-canal models that use number 10 batteries. I got the first aid, for my left ear, 11 years ago—long before I had any vision loss. Handling the tiny batteries was no problem until my vision decreased and I could barely see where to put in a new battery. I tried changing a battery with my eyes closed, but was not successful. Even with my eyes open, I was dropping the tiny batteries on the floor. Eventually I learned to change batteries over a counter or table to minimize the danger of them falling on the floor. Sitting in an upholstered chair to change a battery can lead to the battery falling into a cranny of the chair, making it even harder to find than one that has fallen on the floor.

Dropped or lost batteries can be more than an aggravation—they can be very dangerous to a pet or a young grandchild, who might be attracted to them and swallow them. Even though hearing aid batteries no longer contain mercury and do not need to be recycled, they can cause serious gastric problems if swallowed.

I recently got a new hearing aid for my left ear, this time a behind-the-ear model that uses the large, number 13 battery. When I went to the audiologist to select my new aid, I found that she had already picked out the brand that was easiest in terms of changing batteries. I practiced changing the battery with my eyes closed several times, and I was successful.

At the time I began using the number 13 batteries, my hearing was still at a level that would have allowed me to continue using another small hearing aid that required number 10 batteries, but I wanted to be prepared for both future hearing loss and the need to manipulate the batteries with diminished vision. My new aid is currently set at about the middle of its volume level, so it should last me indefinitely because the audiologist can program the volume to higher levels as time goes on.

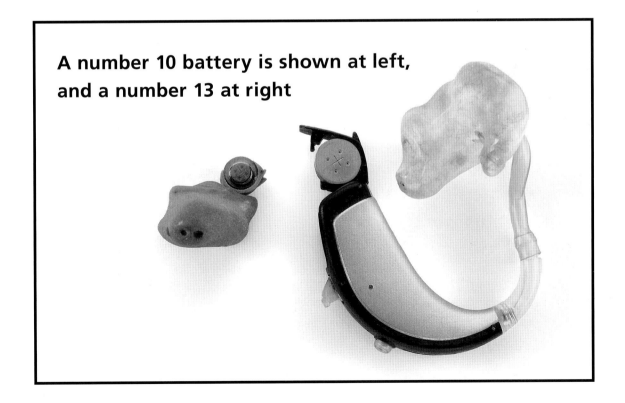

A number 10 battery is shown at left, and a number 13 at right

Are You Lip Reading Without Realizing It?

I was very surprised when my audiologist had me perform tests that showed I was relying heavily on lip reading without even knowing it. First she placed me in a booth with a glass wall dividing us. I was wearing special earphones that allowed me to hear her voice, and I could see her on the other side of the glass wall as she read word after word. As she said each word, I tried to repeat it out loud back to her. She kept a score of how many I got correct. Then I closed my eyes so that I could not see her enunciating the words. I was amazed to learn that I got 92 percent of the words correct when I was watching the audiologist, but only 72 percent correct when I could not see her. These results showed that I was doing a lot of lip reading.

Here are some helpful strategies for dealing with a hearing loss when you also have diminished vision. These ideas were suggested to me by my audiologist, and I have found them very useful.

- Train yourself to listen—try closing your eyes when watching television or chatting with someone, or listen to an audio book.
- Ask people to speak slowly and enunciate clearly.
- Ask people to look directly at you when speaking so that the sound comes directly to you. Even if you can't watch their lips, you should be able to see their body language

and gestures, such as arm waving—valuable cues that will help you understand what the speakers are saying.

- Find the best listening spot in your house of worship by trying different seating locations.

- Use assistive listening devices at movies, theaters, concerts, and other such venues.

- Use a personal amplifier when watching TV.

- In restaurants, ask for a quiet table off to the side, near a wall. Face the wall rather than the room—if you sit facing the room, with all the noise in front of you and a quiet wall behind you, the speaker's voice at your table can become overpowered by all the noise that is also coming right at you from the room. When you face the wall, the loudest sounds will come from the people speaking at your table who are facing you.

Most important of all—**become an advocate for yourself and let others know what you need.**

MY STORY

The Dog Ate My Hearing Aid

Be careful where you put your hearing aids. Even more dangerous to a pet than swallowing a battery is eating an entire hearing aid. If you have a pet, be very careful to place your aids in their container when you remove them from your ears. Dogs and cats are attracted to the hum of a hearing aid that hasn't been turned off, as well as to the scent of wax that may adhere to the inner part of a hearing aid.

Three years ago I carelessly placed my aid on my bedside table. That night, my son's visiting dog became violently ill. I didn't make the connection until a couple of days later, when I realized my aid was hopelessly lost. Fortunately the hearing aid was very small and the dog recovered, but a larger aid could have caused serious internal injuries.

Things turned out just fine for the dog, but I had to spend hundreds of dollars on a new hearing aid.

Use Talking Health Care Products That Announce Your Results

There is a huge variety of specialty products that provide audio as well as visual information. These products can help you remain independent in taking care of personal health care tasks. They are available at low vision stores. Here are just some of the "talking" products available today from low vision stores.

- Blood pressure monitors
- Glucose meters
- Pedometers that announce the numbers of steps you have taken and the total distance traveled

- Scales that speak your weight or that have detachable displays that you can hold as close to your eyes as you need in order to read them

- Thermometers that state your temperature reading

Use Special Products and Tricks in Personal Care

The ideas listed below will help you as you go about your tasks of personal care.

Brushing Teeth

- Use an electric toothbrush that is kept upright in a stand on your vanity. You'll be able to find the toothbrush easily, and electric toothbrushes help you to take good care of your teeth.

- Buy toothpaste in a pump dispenser that stands upright on the counter. This is easier to find than a tube with its tiny cap that can easily disappear when you put it down on your bathroom vanity.

- Solve the problem of getting the toothpaste onto toothbrush bristles that may be difficult to see by putting the toothpaste on your finger, then transferring it to the toothbrush—or, even easier, by putting the toothpaste on your finger, then transferring it directly to your mouth.

Caring for Nails

- Use emery boards instead of nail clippers to keep fingernails and toenails trimmed—you can file by feel, and you won't accidentally cut too much or injure yourself.

- Have a regular pedicure if basic toenail care is difficult for you. Note that home visits by pedicurists are available in some communities. If you would rather not visit a pedicurist for basic toenail maintenance but you have a hard time reaching your toes, try to enlist the help of a friend or relative who will keep your toenails in good condition by filing them with an emery board.

- Visit a podiatrist for nail clipping and to care for foot problems such as ingrown toenails or other foot-related problems, such as corns or calluses. If you are diabetic, this service should be covered by Medicare.

Grooming

- Skip using lipstick, which can be difficult to properly apply, and instead use tinted lip gloss. If you "go outside the lines," it will not be noticeable. Lip glosses and shimmers usually cost less than lipstick, and some brands also act as moisturizing lip balms.

- Use magnifying mirrors for close-work grooming tasks. These are available in many sizes, shapes, and magnification levels. Some are lighted. There are handheld models, models on stands, and wall-mounted models with the magnifiers at the end of swivel arms.

- Use an electric razor for shaving safety.

Bathing and Showering

- Install grab bars in your tub and shower areas. They will help you orient yourself in the shower and will provide a means of support when getting in and out of the shower or tub. For more information on grab bars, see page 95.

- Use a shower bench or transfer bench if you feel unsteady in the shower or if you find it difficult to enter or exit the tub or shower. For more information on these products, see pages 95–97.

PART 2

Using Practical Hints to Make Your Life Easier

IDEAS FOR INDEPENDENT day-to-day living are offered in this section. Some ideas involve using or rearranging things you already have, while others involve getting low-cost products designed for people with vision loss. These products are available at low vision stores, which carry a huge variety of other useful items as well. Most of the products described in this book are available from one or more of the stores that are listed in Appendix A, Suppliers of Low Vision Products. There is space in this book to discuss only a small portion of the many useful products that can be purchased, but most of the stores listed offer catalogs that you can order, either over the phone or by visiting the stores' Web sites. **Order your catalogs today!**

5

Cooking and Eating Using Senses of Touch and Hearing

WOULD YOU GUESS that your sense of touch could become the most important sense when cooking food? You probably would first think of taste, then perhaps smell. You will be surprised by how important your sense of touch will become in compensating for your diminishing sense of sight. Even your sense of hearing will become important in the kitchen.

As you go about your tasks in the kitchen, be aware of activities that are becoming difficult and start thinking about new ways you can do them. Develop the attitude of a creative thinker who is finding solutions to cooking challenges. The ideas in this book will start you along that path. Some of the suggestions in this food section are my own, but most were learned in an inspiring class I took at Vision Loss Resources in Minneapolis. The name of the class is Independent Living Skills, and the ideas presented in it have been gathered from participants over an 18-year period. I am indebted to all of the people who shared their ideas over the years.

Preparing Food

There are simple items available that you can be use to make food preparation easier. These items become useful helpers as you learn the new ways to cook that are described in this chapter. Some useful items are:

- Set of metal measuring cups
- Two sets of metal measuring spoons; the spoons of one set can be bent at right angles to make dippers
- Special paint pens that make permanent raised dots that identify items
- Saucer
- Funnels of various sizes
- Needle-nose pliers or ring opener
- Talking or giant timer
- Towels—one dark, one white
- Cutting boards—one black, one white
- Heavy rubber bands
- Pair of fingered gloves with nonslip silicone grips, such as 'Ove' Glove® gloves

Using Your Sense of Touch in the Kitchen

People with diminished vision often have difficulty identifying items such as measuring cups and spoons or dials on the cooktop and oven. The solution is to use a special paint pen to apply small dots of paint that raise, harden, and become water- and dishwasher-proof. These dots are informally known as "high marks." You will develop your sense of touch by feeling the number of dots on the handles and dials on your appliances.

Paint pens are available at low vision stores. They come in a variety of colors, including black, white, and orange, and the paint adheres to just about any surface, including plastic and metal. One brand of tactile paint pen is the HI-MARK™. The dots are produced by squirting a paint-like substance from the pen onto the surface you want to mark.

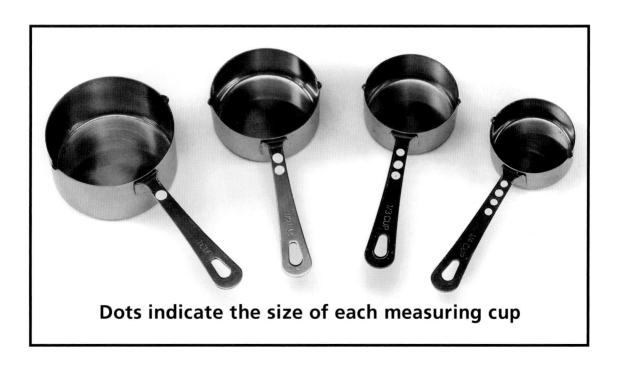

Dots indicate the size of each measuring cup

In order to make sure there is plenty of space on which to place the dots, get metal measuring cups and spoons with long handles and place the dots on the handles close to the cup or spoon so you are able to grasp the ends of the handles. So that you can tell one measuring cup from another, put one dot on the 1-cup measure, two dots on the ½-cup measure, three dots on the ⅓-cup measure, and four dots on the ¼-cup measure. Use the same system on your measuring spoons. To find the measuring cup or spoon you need, pick one up and slide your thumb along the top of the handle to feel the number of dots.

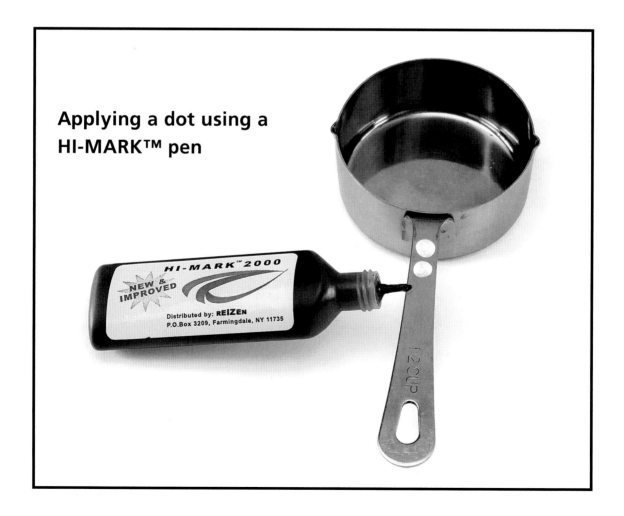

Applying a dot using a HI-MARK™ pen

Ranges, Cooktops, and Ovens—Electric or Gas?

Burners on electric ranges and cooktops are generally safer than gas burners because it is easier to see the color of an electric burner, which becomes redder as it becomes hotter, than it is to see any height of the blue flame on a gas burner. Even a flashlight beam pointed at a gas burner does not make its flame visible, so it can be impossible to even tell, just by looking, whether a low flame is still going or has extinguished. A suggestion is to apply high marks at the settings you generally use. It is recommended that you stick to cooking over low and medium heat, as you don't want to take chances with a high heat that could lead to boilovers. For both gas and electric ovens, it is best to place a high mark at the 350-degree setting and perhaps also at one higher temperature setting, such as 400 degrees, if you often cook at that temperature.

Microwave Cooking

Follow these useful tips when using your microwave oven.

- Buy frozen vegetables in bags rather than in boxes. This way, you can remove just the portion you want, then close the bag and put it back in your freezer for the next use.

- Stir food at the midpoint of its cooking time to ensure that the food is thoroughly cooked or heated.

- Cook bacon in the microwave oven by placing strips between several sheets of paper towels to make thick pads to absorb the fat.

- Use your sense of hearing to listen closely to the number of beeps when you press the buttons to set the cooking time. One extra push of the minute button, for instance, could lead to overcooking, a smoke-filled oven, or worse.

When selecting a new microwave oven, consider looking for a model with some of the following special options.

- A "30 seconds" button, so you can easily set the time for ½, 1½, or 2½ minutes.

- Contrasting display colors, such as black print on a white background or white print on a black background—find the color combination that is easiest for you to see.

- A "talking" feature that prompts you to set the time and that announces cooking time settings, the running cooking time, the current power level, and such phrases as "microwave running," "attend to food," and so forth. High-end models that announce the current time and that have a speech volume control are available at low vision stores.

- A sensor that helps to prevent overcooking or undercooking by determining when the food is ready based on infrared light or by the steam emitted from the food.

- The door handle that works best for you, whether it requires pulling or has a bar or button to push to open the door.

For a review of the accessibility of microwave ovens and other kitchen and laundry appliances, visit the American Foundation™ for the Blind's Web site at www.afb.org and click on "Newsletters." The newsletter *AccessWorld*® offers useful reviews of specific brands and recommendations of specific models.

Making Recipes

Always start by washing your hands—you will be using your fingers in new ways.

When making something in a mixing bowl, first lay out all your ingredients to one side of the bowl. After each ingredient is added, move its container to the other side of the bowl. Then you'll never have to wonder whether or not you have added a particular item. If you are using a white bowl, place a dark towel underneath it for contrast. If you have a dark bowl, use a white towel.

Measuring Ingredients

Your sense of touch again comes into play when you use your measuring cups and spoons. The first thing to do is place a towel on your work space, under your measuring tools and your mixing bowl, cutting board, or other such items to catch drips and spills and to keep bowls and cutting boards from sliding.

If you are working with wet ingredients, keep a saucer handy as a place to put measuring cups and spoons that may be dripping. If you are measuring dry ingredients such as flour or sugar, find the size of measure you want and dip it into the canister. But don't try to use a knife to level the scoopful. You have a much handier instrument—your index finger.

For small amounts of wet and liquid ingredients, use measuring spoons that have been bent to form dippers. If you are unable to see how much of an ingredient is in a measuring spoon, use your finger to level off the top.

Mixing Ingredients

When mixing ingredients by hand, first mix six strokes on one diagonal, then six strokes on the other. Follow this with a few crosswise strokes. When using an electric mixer, always attach the beaters before you plug in the mixer. When you have finished using the mixer, unplug it before removing the beaters. This is an important safety measure.

Cooking on the Range or Cooktop

Here are some handy tips on using senses other than sight to prepare foods on cooktops.

- Rolling boils can be detected in two ways—by hearing the boil or by using your hand, placed a few inches above the pan, to feel the amount of steam that is being produced.

- You can judge whether or not onions have become golden brown by sampling some that have cooled a bit. Both the taste of the onion and its tender texture will let you know.

- When frying foods, place a splatter guard on top of your pan. The guard will prevent hot grease and little pieces of food from flying out of the pan to those hard-to-spot, hard-to-clean places on your cooktop.

Cooking in the Oven

Follow these handy tips when cooking food in the oven.

- Cake batter should be poured into just one spot in the pan (even a Bundt pan), then leveled off, first by quickly sliding the pan on the counter, first from side to side, then away from and toward you. You may finish off the process with a couple of taps of the pan on the counter, as many have been taught.

- Never reach into a hot or heating oven to place a pan on the oven rack or to remove the pan from the rack. Instead, wear your oven-safe gloves, pull the rack out, and place or remove your pan. This is a safety measure to prevent burns.

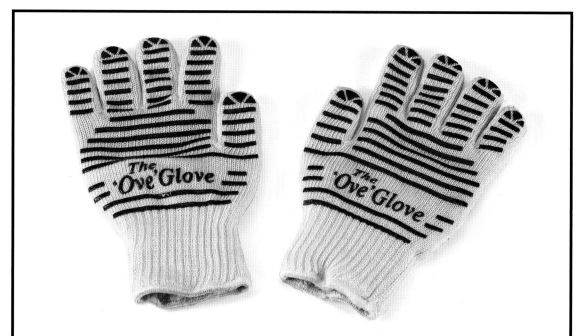

Insulated gloves, such as the 'Ove' Gloves shown here, protect your hands

Using Timers

Many types of timers are available from low vision stores. Set the timer for the amount of time a food is to be cooked or when it is to be checked, and use your sense of hearing to listen for the ring that will tell you the set amount of time has elapsed. Timers range in size from small digital models that are about three inches in height to a dial model that is a huge nine inches in diameter and that has a loud and long ring. There are also timers you can hang around your neck. Check your catalogs to find all the possibilities and choose a model that seems right for you. You may want to try a few different types. Timers don't have to be used just for cooking—you may want to also keep some in other rooms, such as your bedroom to awaken you from a nap.

Using Hearing or Touch to Pour Liquids into a Glass or Cup

Here is a system for pouring hot liquids into glasses or cups. It requires a lot of concentration, so it may take a little practice, but it really works.

- Before you start to pour, make sure the spout of the liquid's container is pointing toward the glass or cup.
- Slowly pour the liquid into the glass or cup.
- Listen to the whooshing sound of the liquid going into the glass or cup.
- When the sound diminishes, the glass or cup is almost full, so prepare to stop pouring.
- When there is no sound, the glass is full, so stop pouring.

For cold liquids, you can place the thumb of your non-pouring hand inside the glass or cup, near the top. Stop pouring when you feel the liquid touch your thumb.

More Tricks of the Trade from Cooks Who Would Not Give Up

- When making coffee, dip your scoop into the coffee, then feel the top of the scoop with your thumb to check the level. If the scoop is too full, use a finger to scrape off the excess coffee.

You can measure out one tablespoon from a stick of butter by using your index finger as a measure, placing it flat, perpendicular to the length of the butter.

It is very difficult to feel most oils that are at room temperature with your finger, and most cooking oils solidify when kept in the refrigerator. Canola oil, however, remains a liquid when stored in the refrigerator—when pouring it into a glass or cup, you will be able to feel the level of the chilled liquid. Canola oil is one of the more healthful oils, too.

Spray measuring cups with vegetable oil spray—inside and outside—so food won't stick to the cups.

Use oil sprays over the sink so you don't get any on the floor and slip.

Use a black or dark cutting board to slice light foods, such as onions, and a white cutting board to slice dark foods, such as cooked meat.

Marinate meat in a zipped plastic bag.

Find which side of a milk carton to open by sliding your finger along the top to feel which side has the crease.

To open cans with pull tabs, use needle-nose pliers or just stick a spoon under the tab.

Cook Large Batches

To reduce that amount of time you need to spend cooking, make multiple portions of favorite meals and freeze individual servings for quick, handy meals that you can heat in the microwave oven.

Use Large Print and Specialty Cookbooks

Many cookbooks are available in large print versions that are easier to read than the regular editions. You can find the books in many libraries and in some bookstores. Some online booksellers, such as Amazon (www.amazon.com) and Large Print Books (www.largeprintbooks.com), carry a wide variety of large print titles.

If you have a medical condition that restricts your diet, nutrition becomes even more important. Take the time and effort to find foods that you enjoy. Consult a specialty cookbook. Cookbooks are available for diabetic, cardiac, renal, and gluten-free diets—in fact, no matter what dietary restrictions you have, there is probably at least one cookbook that will work for you. Some of these cookbooks come in large print editions.

MY STORY

Packaging Takeout Food for the Freezer

I have food restrictions imposed by a medical condition. Two years ago, after six months of steady weight loss, my doctor diagnosed celiac disease, which is an intolerance to gluten. The treatment is to eat no wheat, oats, rye, or barley. Although gluten-free foods are becoming more commonly available in food stores, I wasn't satisfied with the frozen dinners I found. Then I discovered that many Indian and Thai foods were gluten free, and I found excellent local restaurants specializing in these cuisines.

Now I purchase, for takeout, a selection of entrées from these restaurants and freeze them for quick meals that are ready after four minutes in the microwave oven. Before freezing them, I divide each entrée into two or three portions, as the servings are so large.

Round, square, or rectangular? I use different shapes of plastic storage containers for different items, based on the main ingredient of each dish. The dishes are basically rice or noodles plus meat. I store chicken dishes in round containers, beef dishes in rectangular containers, and shrimp dishes in square containers.

I place each container shape in a different section of the freezer shelf—left, middle, and right. When I decide

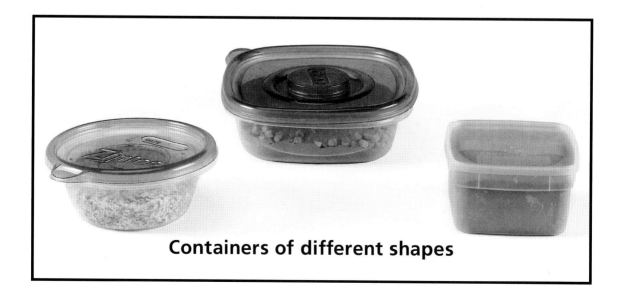

Containers of different shapes

which one I want, I can pull it out of the freezer without even looking. Then I open the container's lid slightly to allow steam to escape while the dish is cooking, place the container in the microwave oven, and close the oven door. Next, I find the knob for the one-minute button, and I punch it four times. Once the dish is heated, I dump the food into a plastic bowl so I don't have to worry about spills while I'm eating, and I enjoy a meal that has been no work to prepare and that is tastier and often cheaper than any frozen dinner I could buy in a store.

Using Identification Techniques When Eating

These tips will make it easier to find what you are looking for when eating, making mealtimes more enjoyable.

- Use color contrast to help locate items at your place setting. Put dark dishes on white placemats, and light dishes on dark placemats.

- Use colored or patterned drinking glasses rather than transparent glasses.

- Avoid plates with patterns, which can be visually confusing when you are trying to locate your food.

- Use tactile markers to help distinguish items such as salt, pepper, and sauce containers. These items can be wrapped in rubber bands or marked with raised dots.

- Identify foods by exploring your plate with your fork, or ask someone to describe the location of different items—what's at the top, bottom, right, and left on the plate. Or use the clock-face method to describe each food's position—for example, that peas are at three o'clock, meat at six o'clock.

- Position your plate so that the meat is nearest to you, as this is the easiest position for cutting.

Going Out to Eat

Eating at a restaurant need not be frustrating. Follow these tips, and enjoy your meal in confidence.

Seating

- Ask for a table or booth where the lighting is the brightest.

- If you are troubled by glare, ask to be seated where glare is not present or where blinds can be drawn.

- If you are hard of hearing, also ask for a table where the level of noise is low. See page 53 for more tips on choosing where to sit in a restaurant when you have hearing loss.

Menus

- Bring along a pen light or a flashlight that's placed in a Flashlite Friend to help you read the menu. See pages 32–34 and 208 for information on this handy device.

Bring along a magnifying glass, as it may enable you to read the menu.

If you are unable to read the menu, ask your dining companion to read it out loud for you—this can prompt some fun discussions.

If you are dining alone and are unable to read the menu, ask the server to read the sections, such as appetizers, main courses, or desserts, that interest you.

You can avoid the menu entirely by asking the waiter for the specials of the day or for his or her personal recommendations.

Eating

Decide on your selections before you leave home by checking the restaurant's Web site to look for a posted menu; if it's available online, print it on white paper, study it in good light, and choose what you want to order in advance.

Select finger food or easy-to-eat dishes that don't require a lot of cutting and that are easy to distinguish on a plate.

Ask that meats be cut in the kitchen.

Bring out your Flashlite Friend to point its light onto your plate.

And laugh when you completely miss what you're aiming for with your fork and try to spear the table instead.

6

Organizing Your Living Space

HAVE YOU ACCUMULATED all sorts of stuff over the years? If you have lived in the same place for a long time, it will be especially difficult to follow the common advice to sort through all these possessions and keep only what you really want and use. If you have recently downsized to a smaller place, this task won't be as hard as it is for someone who continues to live in the same house he or she has occupied for 42 years, like me.

In addition to organizing the things where you live, you will want to analyze your living quarters to make sure there are no safety hazards, such as obstacles you might not see. You can also maximize the visibility of large objects such as furniture. Some low vision organizations make home visits to check the safety of your home and offer help in making it safer.

Sorting and Storing or Tossing

For people with declining vision, it is especially important to get started on downsizing and organizing right away, before it becomes more difficult to see what you are dealing with. Another reason for doing the weeding now is that, if you don't do it yourself, someone else will end up doing it later. Is that what you'd want?

Before you get to work on organizing what you have, get rid of anything you don't need. Sort through your closets, drawers, and so forth and toss or give away the things you do not use. You would be wasting time by finding places for things you really don't want.

Giving Away Clothing

If you have "vintage" or valuable designer clothing that is in good condition, you could take it to a consignment shop, but ask your children first if they want any of these items. In many communities, there are charitable organizations that will pick up clothing and, sometimes, household items that you no longer want. The point is to clear out your closets and bureau drawers of things you no longer use so that you will have fewer things to search through when looking for what you want to wear that day.

Looking at Mementos

When you go through your possessions, set aside things you think your children or other loved ones would like to have. It would be even better to have one of them help you with this task, because seeing precious things that have been stashed away can be an emotional experience. What may seem a difficult undertaking can be turned into a special time with a child when you share with him or her the history of an item that means a lot to you.

Organize those photos that may be lumped together in a box or stuffed into a drawer. You might want to go through them with family members and tell them a bit of family history or remember happy occasions together. Have your favorite photos enlarged and put in simple frames for yourself and the people pictured in the photos. Inexpensive frames are available at drug and discount stores.

Perhaps the most difficult task is to sort through letters and cards you have been keeping. It helps to be in the right mood—this is a very sentimental task, but it's one that is best done by you.

——————————— MY STORY ———————————
History for My Daughter and My Farewell to "Dating" Dresses

My daughter learned a lot about me when I told her my history with each dress in an old closet in the basement.

I hadn't looked at them in 20 years and dreaded seeing the condition they were in after all that time of improper storage. Without the support of my daughter, I could never have gone through that closet. Actually, she was the one who took the dresses down from the clothes rod, one by one. I was not up to the task because I hated to think how my precious dresses might look. Each elicited a story, mostly about a special date with her father, occasions that remained vivid memories. She was enthralled to hear about the early days of her dad and me, but remembering those happy times was a very emotional and nostalgic experience for me, especially because my husband had died only a few weeks earlier. It was also sad to see that the dresses were now full of holes. My daughter convinced me that there was no point in hanging onto them and that we should take care of matters then and there. I made my sad farewells and, a short time later, the dresses were gone. She had taken care of their disposal out of my view, for which I was thankful.

Putting Everything in Its Place

As you proceed with the weeding, you can start finding places for everything you are going to keep.

Finding Things in Drawers

Try to keep clothing you use frequently, such as underwear and socks, in an upper, easily reached drawer of a bureau, where it will be less difficult to reach and see what's in the drawer. It can become almost impossible to see items in a bottom drawer because lighting is poor near the floor. For me, even a flashlight does not help. If there is furniture in your bedroom with high drawers, but a partner with better vision is using them, try to make a trade of a couple of drawers so you will be better able to see what is inside.

Boxes are the secret to organizing and finding things in drawers. Be on the lookout for boxes that will fit inside your drawers. Shoe boxes work well for small items—you can put particular colors of underwear or socks in them. You can even use a tissue box. Cut the top so that you can fold sections of it to the inside edges of the box, and secure them in place with heavy tape.

If you find a particular kind of sock you like or an undergarment that fits just right, you might think about stocking up on that item so you don't have so much trouble distinguishing one color or style from another.

Arranging Shirts and Pants in Closets

If you're like me and have a plain, old-fashioned closet with clothes rods, but no fancy organizers, these tricks should be helpful, and they don't cost a cent. Of course, the first step is to get rid of all those clothes you haven't worn in years. Then you can organize what you have. Here are several ideas.

- Use white garments to separate the various colors of tops and shirts in your wardrobe. The colors of my clothes are organized in my closet in this way: white, pink, white, black, white, blue, white, brown.

- When certain items go only with each other, hang them side by side.

- Leave the white paper on hangers from the dry cleaners to provide color contrast—that makes it easier to see what is on the hanger. You can also get colored plastic hangers and hang blue tops on blue hangers, brown on brown, and so forth.

- If none of the above methods works for you, try the "safety pin method." This system can be used for all types of clothing, from shirts and pants to jackets and dresses. Use small brass safety pins to identify clothing items by fastening a certain number of pins in the back labels or side tabs of each color of clothing item. The number of pins attached to a garment identifies its color. Because black is the most common color, you might want to leave black clothes free of safety pins—that will be their code. Here is an example of the system.

Black—no pin
White—one pin
Brown—two pins
Navy—three pins
Green—four pins

■ Shoes can also be difficult to identify by color, especially if you have the same style in more than one color. You can use the same color coding system, but use clothes pins instead of safety pins. For example, you might clip together a pair of brown shoes with one clothes pin, and a pair of navy shoes with two pins.

Organizing Earrings and Other Jewelry

If you have lots of earrings, pins, necklaces, or other jewelry, sort out the things you wear frequently and organize them in a plastic container with transparent compartments. For my earrings and small pins, I bought an inexpensive organizer, shown here, at a craft store. It has fourteen small compartments in two rows. Each row locks separately, and each compartment has a tight lid that won't open until the

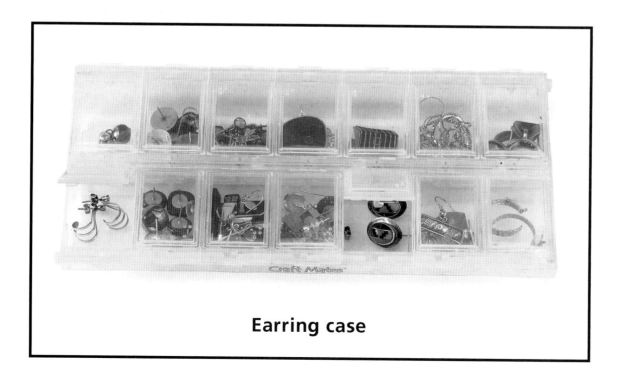

Earring case

row is unlocked by pushing a little button on the side. One or two pairs of earrings fit into each compartment. Pick out your favorite earrings and organize them using a system that makes sense to you, with your favorites on the end compartments.

This is also the time to start practicing putting earrings in your pierced ears without looking in the mirror.

Weeding Your Medicine Cabinet

Start organizing your medicine cabinet by disposing of items you no longer use and by throwing out medications that have passed their expiration dates. You do not want any outdated medicine in your cabinets. Keep your bottles of pills and other medicines and supplements that you take regularly, such as the AREDS formula, in a large plastic zip bag so they are handy when you are filling your pill containers. Over-the-counter medicines that you take occasionally may be kept in your bathroom cabinet along with lotions, hair and nail care products, and other personal care products. Arrange items in a way that makes sense to you so you will know where each item is kept.

Organizing Your Kitchen

Here are some ideas on organizing food in your kitchen cupboards, refrigerator, and freezer that have worked for other people. You can devise your own systems that will work for you. This is a good place to use your imagination to think of ways to adapt the arrangement of your canned goods and other food items.

Identifying and Arranging Canned Goods

Some canned goods are easy to distinguish from others. For instance, it's not difficult to tell a can of soup from a can of tuna. But identifying the kind of soup that's in the can is another matter entirely. Here are some tricks you can use, all involving the sense of touch.

- Rubber bands: No band for your favorite soup—let's say tomato. One rubber band around, say, chicken noodle soup, and two around vegetable beef. You can use the same system for canned vegetables.

- Instead of rubber bands, you can use pennies taped to the tops of cans.

- A third option is to write, in large letters, the name of each can's contents on an index card. Wrap each card around the correct can and hold it in place with a rubber band. This is a handy system because the cards can be used over and over.

- A fourth option is to place magnets with large letters or vegetable shapes on cans.

If you don't have many varieties of canned goods, you can identify the cans by placing them in assigned locations on the shelf.

Organizing Food in the Refrigerator and Freezer

If you live with other people, designate one shelf in the refrigerator for any special food you may like or need for a special diet. Others in your household may have their own shelves, too. Arrange your items so that each one has a regular place. Use the same system in the freezer—everything in its place. See pages 73–75 for ideas on storing refrigerated or frozen foods in containers.

Filling Prescriptions and Organizing Medications

By the time in your life that you have a loss of vision, you probably also have other medical conditions that require medication. Making sure you have the pills you need and remembering to take them at the correct time each day can consume a lot of time. Getting medications organized can be a difficult and frustrating task, and at some point you may want to get some help.

Filling Prescriptions

To save a lot of time and trouble in getting refills, ask your doctor to write each prescription for a three-month period, if paying for the larger quantity will fit in your budget. See if your pharmacy offers large print copies of the bottle labels. Some pharmacies use easy-to-read labels placed on flat bottles. Use the pharmacy that best suits your needs.

Cutting Pills in Half

If you need to cut pills in half, you can get a handy pill cutter with a built-in magnifier at some low vision stores. A plastic lid over the blade keeps the cut pieces from flying about. Still, this is a job you may want someone else to do. Some pharmacists will cut the pills for you.

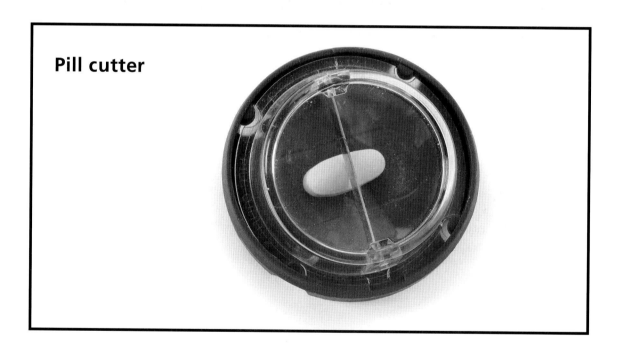

Pill cutter

Did I Take My Pills? Using Pill Organizers

Solve the problem of remembering to take your medications at the correct times each day by using pill organizers. Organizers are available at drugstores and at low vision stores.

- If you take meds only in the morning and evening, it is handy to use two seven-compartment organizers, each with a slot for each day of the week. Get different-colored organizers for morning and evening.

- If you take meds three or four times a day, an organizer with four rows and twenty-eight compartments would allow you to get all your meds for the week in one container.

- There are many different sizes, colors, and configurations of organizers—there's even one with an alarm system. Decide what would work best for you.

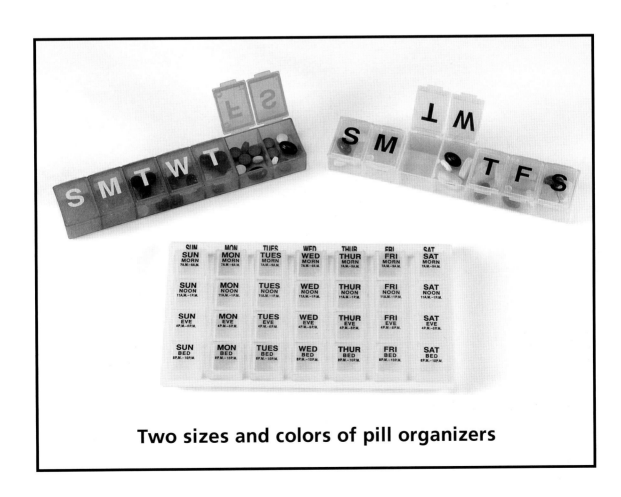

Two sizes and colors of pill organizers

Avoid Bouncing Pills When Filling a Pill Organizer

It is easy to drop pills on the floor while transferring them from the bottles to the right compartment in the organizer. Stop the spill by sitting at a table and placing a large tray under the bottles and the organizer. If you drop a pill it will land on the tray, and the sides of the tray should keep it from rolling or bouncing onto the floor. Begin with all the bottles placed to one side of the organizer. As you finish putting each bottle's pills in their compartments, close that bottle and move it to the other side. This way, you won't have to wonder if you have already used that bottle.

––––––––––––––––––– **MY STORY** –––––––––––––––––––

Saturday Night Ritual of Picking Up Pills

Every Saturday night my husband filled his pill containers. And every Saturday night, at least one tiny pill would slip from his hand and end up on the floor. He had good eyes, but he didn't have the agility or strength to get down on the floor to find the pill. It was up to me, the one with the poor vision, to get down on my hands and knees and look where he was pointing. Part of the routine involved getting a flashlight so I'd have a chance of finding the pill. I always eventually found it, but often it was far from where he thought it had landed. This was our ritual until he became ill and had to go to a nursing home. I wish we had thought of the tray trick earlier.

Doing Laundry

People with diminished vision face two big problems when it comes to doing laundry—getting the right amount of detergent into the washer and matching up socks from the dryer. The following ideas will help with these tasks.

Measuring the Detergent in the Cap

Here are two ways to get the correct amount of detergent into your laundry load.

- As you pour liquid detergent, place the index finger of the hand holding the cap inside the cap to the level you want. Stop pouring the detergent when you feel the liquid on the tip of your finger.

- For either liquid or powder detergent, use a measuring cup instead of the cap.

Matching Socks

Even those with good vision can find it very difficult to pair up socks as they come out of the dryer. Here are two tricks to make this a snap.

- One way to eliminate the problem is to have all identical socks—one style, one color—so that no matching is needed. Once you find a style you like, buy multiple pairs, and you will not have to worry about matching up socks again.

- If you have a variety of socks, use large safety pins to fasten pairs together at the heel as you take off the socks at night. Color code the socks by using two or more pins for colors other than black or white. If you do laundry for others, be sure that they follow this system as well.

Have a Spot-Finder Friend

If you live with someone, make an agreement that he or she will always tell you when you have a spot on your clothing. This will be a great service to you, as spots can be almost impossible to see. A buddy system with a housemate or friend can prevent you from going around with embarrassing spots on your clothing. This will work for toothpaste around your mouth, lipstick on your teeth, or shaving cream under your ear, too.

Finding and Removing Spots from Clothing

When you find out about a spot on your clothing, try to wash it out right away. As an extra precaution, mark the spot with a safety pin and pretreat that area before you place the garment in the washer. For items that must be dry cleaned, mark spots with pins to identify the problems that need special treatment.

Ironing

The best idea is to avoid ironing by buying wrinkle-free clothes, but if you do need to iron, follow these safety precautions.

- Use a paint pen to place high marks on the iron settings.
- Place the ironing board next to a heatproof kitchen counter.
- Put the iron on the counter, not on the ironing board, while you prepare to iron or need to set the iron down to rearrange an item.
- Pour water into the iron through a funnel.
- Never grope around trying to find a hot iron. Instead, lightly run your hand along the cord to find it. As your hand gets close to the iron, you should be able to feel its heat. Stop before you accidentally touch the hot face of the iron.
- Use your hands to determine where wrinkles are.
- Iron in one direction so there will be no wrinkles from dragging the iron back over the clothing.

Safe Passage Through Your Space

Good balance is needed even when walking in your own home, where most accidents occur. See pages 41–43 for ideas on how to improve your balance. Don't trip and fall in your own living space. Try to identify any hazards that could block your way, and move furniture to clear any narrow passageways. If there is a vision loss resource center in your community, call to see if it offers a home evaluation that will spot possible obstacles and hazards and help you find a safer way to arrange your furniture.

Avoid Tripping on Area Rugs

Loose rugs pose a danger for tripping when they can't be seen, especially if you've developed a shuffling walk and may hit the rug with your toe, resulting in a fall. It is the best policy to remove area rugs.

Climbing Stairs

Follow these guidelines when walking up or down stairs.

- Always use the handrail, but consider it a support only—not an indication that you are at the last step. Some rails end before you get there.

- Know the number of steps in the stairs you use every day, and count as you go up and down so you will know where you are.

- If you have a weak leg, lead with the "bad" leg when going down and the "good" leg when going up. Bring your second leg to the same step once the first is firmly in place. For the next step, lead with the same leg you used before—do not alternate legs. You can remember this rule by thinking of the "bad" leg as "going down to hell" and the "good" leg as "going up to heaven."

Bathtub and Shower Safety

Most home accidents occur in the bathroom. Bathing and using the toilet require good strength and balance. Features that can help to keep you safe include:

■ Grab bars near the toilet and in the bathtub and shower

■ Transfer bench or shower chair

■ Nonskid bathtub and shower floor mats

■ Commode or raised toilet seat

■ Reverse door swing, in which the door swings out of, rather than into, the bathroom—this provides more

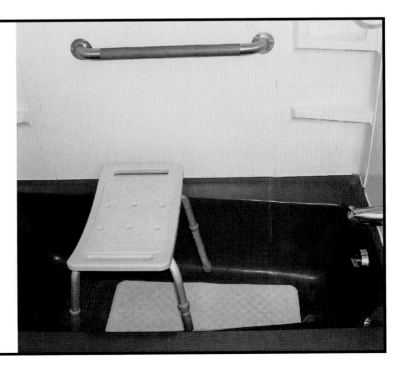

A lightweight shower bench fits inside the tub or shower stall; note the grab bar

space in the bathroom, and the door won't be blocked if someone slips or falls in the bathroom

Use a shower bench if you can step into the shower, but feel unsteady standing up. In the photo, note the rubber mat on the floor of the tub and the grab bar shown in the photo on the previous page. These are also important safety features.

A transfer bench is used by people who cannot safely step into the tub. The legs of the bench are on the outside of tub. One starts by sitting on the part of the seat that is outside the tub, then scooting across the seat until he or she is inside the tub. There are suction cups on the inside legs to prevent the bench from slipping. With the addition

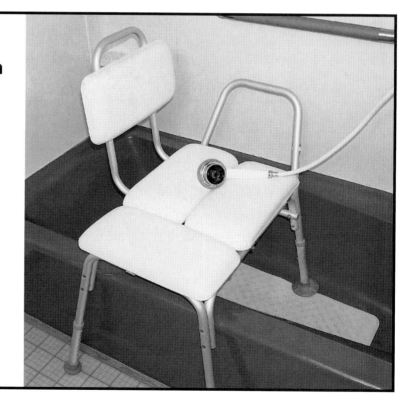

Note the bench legs outside of the tub—you scoot across

of a handheld shower, it is never necessary to stand up in the shower.

It often becomes difficult to sit down and get up from the toilet, especially if one's leg muscles have become weak. There are no arms, as there are on a chair, to push against to help yourself arise. A commode with arms is the answer. In the style shown in the photo, no installation is required, and its height is adjustable in one-inch increments.

A commode with arms that fit over the toilet

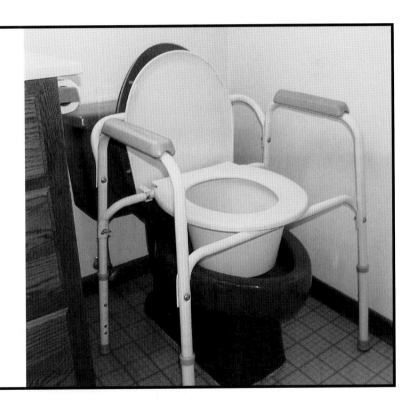

These benches and commodes are available from medical equipment and supply stores. If it is a medical necessity that you use these products, the cost may be covered by health insurance, depending on your plan.

Using the Telephone

It is very dangerous to rush to answer the phone, so phones should be in convenient locations. It would be ideal to have a phone in every room, and this is possible with a cordless system for which you can buy extra handsets.

If the phone jack is far away, sometimes the only way to have a phone in a handy place is to run a phone line along the floor. If this absolutely cannot be avoided, cover the line with heavy shipping tape or masking tape so you will not trip on the loose cord.

Battling Public Doorways

Unfamiliar public doorways can cause frustration. Here are some tips on dealing with them.

- In public places, fire codes require that all doors open to the outside so that people inside a burning building can escape by pushing the door to go outside. This means that you must always PULL the door to enter a public building and PUSH the door to go out.

- Note that a regular door is required to be placed next to a revolving door.

7

Finding
Hard-to-Spot Things

DO THINGS VANISH after you have set them down
somewhere? Is the control button on an appliance
impossible to locate? Are you not able to plug in an
appliance because you can't see the holes in the receptacle
or you can't make the plug fit into the holes?

These are all stressful situations that happen throughout
the day. If you feel like screaming or crying, or maybe
laughing, go ahead—it might make you feel less frustrated.
When you've let off the steam, realize that you can still
do these everyday tasks, but that you will do them in a
different way that will probably take a little longer. Again,
your sense of touch can come to your rescue.

Using Tactile Bumps and Marks to Identify Objects

Small, raised, plastic "bumps" are among the most useful things in my everyday life. Available at low vision stores, these bumps adhere to most surfaces, and they make it possible to find all sorts of things by touch.

Two types of bumps are available. The first are round or square raised bumps that are flat on the bottom, with strong adhesive that attaches to all sorts of surfaces. They come in a variety of sizes, colors, and materials. Besides raised plastic bumps that come in three sizes and colors from white to fluorescent to clear, there are flat stick-ons made of felt, velour, or cork. They come in darker colors than the plastic bumps and provide different textures to the touch. By using a variety of sizes, colors, and textures, you can distinguish things such as such as different buttons on a remote control or special keys on a computer keyboard. For example, I've marked the "delete" key of my computer keyboard with a flat brown stick-on, and the "tab" key is marked with a round raised orange bump. The cost of the bumps is minimal. They come in packs of 10 to 40, depending on the size and material of the bump.

The other type of mark bump is a raised dot made with a pen on surfaces where permanent dots are needed or where adhesive dots will not stick. These raised dots are useful on such items as metal measuring cups and stove dials. See pages 63–64 for a description on using them.

As the years have gone by, I've added the adhesive-backed plastic bumps to more and more items. In my kitchen, I use them on the dishwasher's power button and on the microwave oven's "one minute" and power level buttons. On the TV remote control I have bumps on the power, volume, and "channel up" buttons. Meanwhile, I've used the paint pens to create high marks on my VCR remote control and to draw raised lines on my coffee carafe at the levels I frequently use.

Bumps and high marks can be placed on any number of items—telephone buttons, computer power switches, radio faceplates to mark dial positions of favorite stations, telephones, calculator buttons, keys, dishwashers, clothes

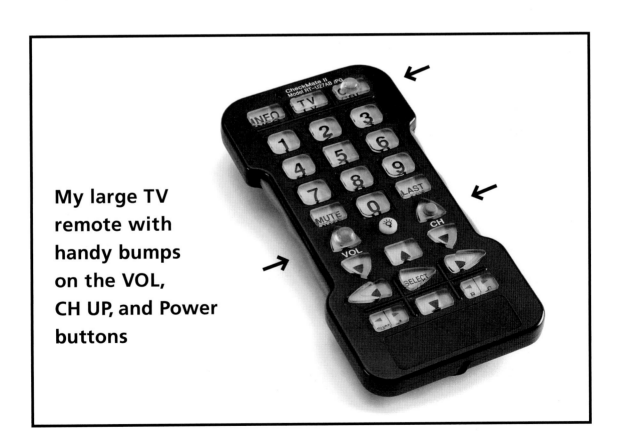

My large TV remote with handy bumps on the VOL, CH UP, and Power buttons

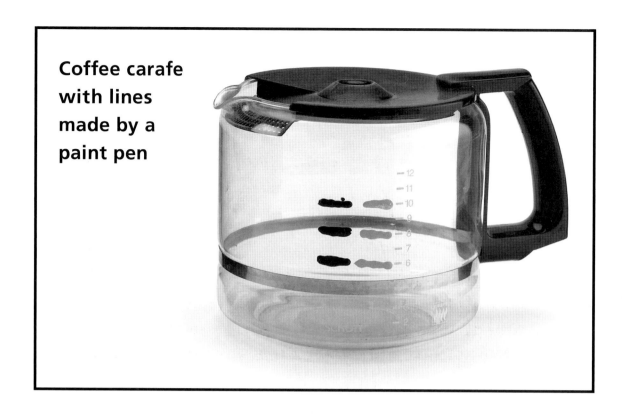

Coffee carafe with lines made by a paint pen

washers, remote controls, and other items you want to recognize by touch. Analyze your own needs, then get busy marking your problem items.

Using White Reflective Tape for Contrast on Dark Objects

Shiny white tape can make it easier to spot items such as a cordless phone, a hearing aid case, and purse pockets. This photo shows the case for my distance-glasses at left, and the case for my reading glasses at right. I can tell them apart because the tape on the distance-glasses case is at an angle. I use black cases for maximum contrast against the white tape. At the bottom of the photo is a hearing aid case that has been taped with two narrow strips so it can be easily spotted when sitting on a counter.

Trying to find something in a purse can be like looking into a deep, black hole. Avoid a purse that has one big pocket, and instead get one that has two or three main compartments and some little pockets in at least one of the compartments. Then figure out what goes in each section, and stick to your plan. I have a purse with side-by-side pockets—one for my cell phone and one for my tiny wallet, which is about two inches by three inches. I've placed reflective tape around the tops of each pocket so I can see where they are. There are other little pockets for pens, cards, and other small items, too. I always put keys in the small outside pocket. My flashlight goes in the medium compartment along with tissues and shopping lists.

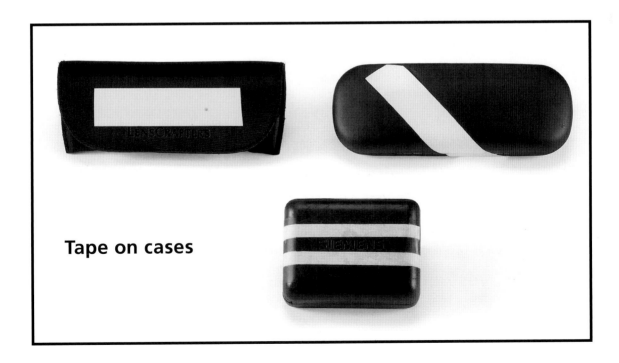

Tape on cases

Can't See Numbers on Your Cell Phone? Try a Jitterbug®

As more and more features have been added to cell phones, the phones themselves have become smaller in size and more difficult to use. Some models are so thin that it is difficult to even spot the tiny phone in a purse or on a counter.

Yet cell phones are useful to people with low vision—for use in emergency situations and to bring along when you are out. Some people no longer have a landline phone and rely entirely on cell phones. But what good are they if you can't read the numbers on the keypad or see the display?

A Jitterbug phone is the answer. They require no contract, and low monthly fees are available. They come in two models, "Dial" and "OneTouch."

Features of the Dial model include:

- Flip-top design that makes the phone 4 inches tall, 2¼ inches wide, and 1 inch deep when closed, so it won't get lost at the bottom of a purse or pocket
- Light feature that is activated when the phone is charging, making it easy to spot
- Large, backlit, bright, easy-to-see buttons on full keypad
- Simple "yes" and "no" action buttons—no confusing icons

- Option to simply press "0" to reach a live Jitterbug operator who will look up and dial a number for you

- Large text on screen

- Personal phone list stored on the phone with easy access

- Hearing-aid compatibility, with padded earpiece that also reduces outside noise

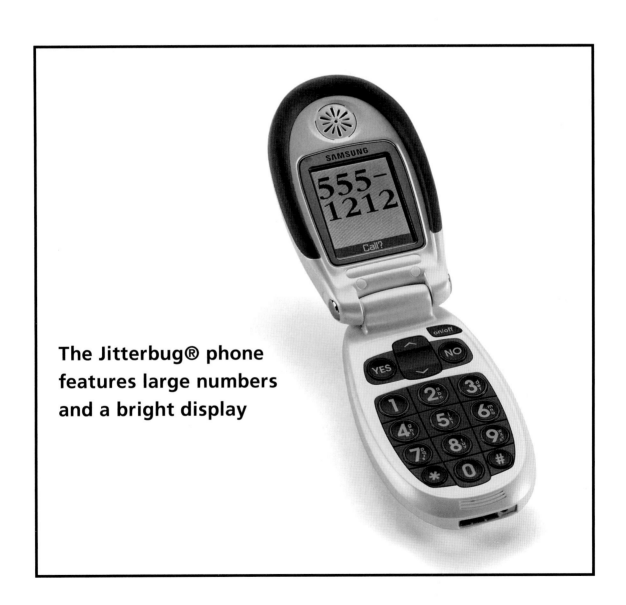

The Jitterbug® phone features large numbers and a bright display

- Audible dial tone

- Convenient, no-mistake volume control

- Comfortable fit, both in your hand and around your ear

- Easy-to-use speakerphone

- Option to update your phone list and features online via your personal, secure Jitterbug Web page—do it yourself, ask a friend, or Jitterbug will do it for you

Features of the OneTouch model include:

- Three large, backlit, easy-to-see and easy-to-feel buttons instead of a keypad

- Operator assistance at the push of the top button—a Jitterbug operator will dial numbers you request

- Middle, direct-dial button that is personally set for you by the company—you can have this button set to call a friend, home, a towing company, or any other person or place you wish

- Immediate, one-touch access to 911 via the bottom button

- **Simple "yes" and "no" action buttons—no confusing icons**

For both phone models, two service plans are available, pay-as-you-go and monthly "anytime, anywhere" minutes ranging from 30 to 800 minutes. No contract is required. Payment can be made automatically by credit card or by writing a monthly check. To order, go to www.jitterbug. com or see Appendix A for contact information.

Writing with a Bold Pen— and Finding It Later

Reading one's own writing becomes more and more difficult as sight diminishes. At first it is easy to read what you write with a pencil, but eventually you can make out only writing done in ink. Then even writing done in black ink can be tough to read. Felt-tip pens provide a darker line and are readily available in many types of stores. If you require an even darker, bolder line, the answer is a Sanford 20/20® pen, available at low vision stores. The ink just flows out of the pen, and the writing is dark and easy to read. The pen is white and its cap is black, so there is good color contrast at both ends, but the pen can still be hard to spot in a jar or box of other pens. You can put a heavy rubber band around the top of the pen to help identify it. If you are still using other pens, put different colors of rubber bands around the tops to help find the pen you want.

Getting Large-Faced or Talking Clocks and Watches

You may find yourself able to see your clock or the watch on your wrist, but not be able to read the time on the dials or digital display. You can buy clocks and watches with very large faces, or you can get a talking clock or watch— all available from low vision stores. Back in the 1980s talking cube clocks were an innovation. Similar clocks are made today, along with many other styles including talking alarm clocks and clock radios.

MY STORY

Grumpy Is Still Talking

My mother had an early cube clock, shown in the photo. She nicknamed it "Grumpy" because of its gruff male voice. When my children were small, they loved pushing the button on the front of the clock to hear the time. When I recently decided I needed a talking clock, I put new batteries in the old clock and pushed the button. After having been idle for 19 years, Grumpy loudly announced the time in that same old gruff voice.

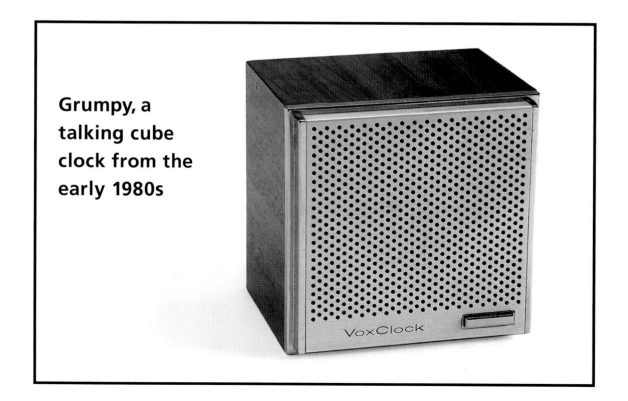

Grumpy, a talking cube clock from the early 1980s

Setting Thermostats

Thermostats can be very difficult to see. You can use high mark dots on a couple of temperature settings or, if a tactile marking isn't possible on your type of thermostat, you can try using nail polish to paint a bright line at your favorite settings. You might want to install a large circular thermostat that has big numbers instead.

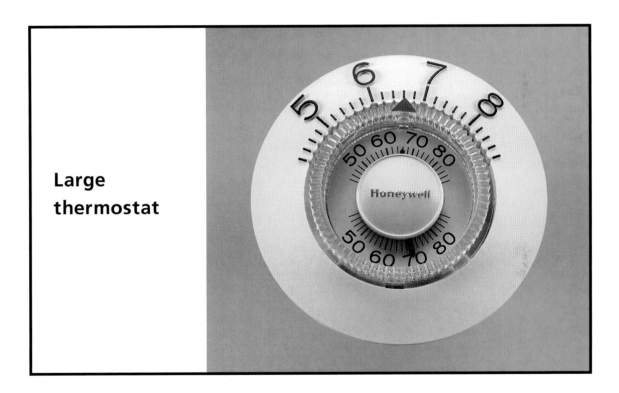

Large thermostat

Making Furniture, Steps, and Light Switches Visible

Here are some ideas on how to make common household items easier to navigate.

Arrange furniture to provide for an easy route around the room.

Put white doilies on the arms and backs of dark-colored chairs.

Put contrasting throw pillows on the sofa.

Cover coffee tables and side tables with bright fabric or something white—whatever will contrast with the flooring color.

Place a bright tablecloth or centerpiece on the dining room or kitchen table.

Use night lights or dimmed lights in hallways, bathrooms, and other rooms you may go into during the night.

Have a beacon by your bed, such as a radio with a dim light—or whatever light it takes to be able to find your way back to bed if you get up during the night. Keep a flashlight, housed in a Flashlite Friend, on your night table.

Mark the first and last steps of your stairs with safety tape or tread strips to make them easier to see.

Use light switch faceplates in colors that contrast with the colors of the walls.

Put contrasting-colored knobs on cupboard doors and dresser drawers.

Have a readily available light at the entrance to each room. If there is no light switch by the door, consider adding a lamp that you can turn on by clapping your hands.

Plugging Cords into Receptacles

To avoid having to bend over or even crawl around the floor trying to find receptacles, get power surge strips with cords that are long enough to allow you to place the strips in convenient places, such as on a side table.

Follow these tips for plugging items into power surge strips.

- Find the wide prong of each plug. Mark that side of the plug with a high mark from a paint pen.

- Find the top end of the power strip—the end nearest the cord that plugs into the receptacle. Position the strip flat on the table, with the top end facing away from you.

- Feel the receptacle to find the side on which the holes with the wide slots are located. Mark the wide side with high marks.

- Using your non-dominant hand, find the receptacle holes. To hold the place, put the pad of your index finger on one side and the pad of your middle finger on the other.

- Using your dominant hand, insert the plug at the end of the cord into the power strip's receptacle.

Finding a Keyhole and Inserting the Key

This is such a foolproof method that it works even when it's dark and you don't know where the lock is on the door.

- Find the key you want on the key ring. Hold it upright in your dominant hand. If the key has ridges on both sides it may be a bit tricky to figure out which way the key should be turned to go into the lock. If there are ridges on only one side of the key, that means that the flat part of the key is the bottom.

- Slide your hand around the door to find the lock.

- Using your finger, find the hole for the key and insert your thumbnail into it.

- Place the key next to your thumbnail.

- Remove your thumbnail from the lock as you slide in the key.

- Turn the key and the doorknob, and open the door.

PART 3

Arranging Your Affairs and Using Assistive Technology

FINANCIAL AND LEGAL aspects of your life are covered in the first chapter of this section. It is easy to push aside the tasks involved in taking care of these personal affairs, but they should be a part of your strategies in preparing for the future. That future can be enriched and expanded by using assistive technology. Chapter 9 discusses its usefulness by describing adaptive products in audio, video, and computer categories.

8

Dealing with Financial, Personal, and Legal Affairs

HELPFUL WAYS TO DEAL with the challenges of managing day-to-day finances are available. Simple aids, credit cards, and banking services can help reduce the huge frustration that may come when we try to do some things that once had been so routine, such as writing a check. Careful planning for managing longer-term legal and financial affairs is also very important. Preparation of legal documents—a will or trust, a health care directive, and a power of attorney—will ensure that your wishes are known and carried out.

Handling Bill Paying and Bank Accounts

Writing checks and keeping a check register can be very difficult for people with macular disease, but there are a variety of ways to make these tasks easier.

Paying Bills Automatically

You can arrange to have your recurring monthly bills, such as gas, electric, telephone, and mortgage bills, paid via automatic deductions from your checking account. Try to arrange to have them paid on a date a few days after your Social Security and other regular deposits, such as a pension, are available in your account. You can still get printed statements from the various companies for these bills in the mail, but they will be marked DO NOT PAY.

Writing Checks

Large print checks, which are about 8 inches across and 3¾ inches high, are available at most banks. They usually have bold black raised lines, and the background is yellow to help reduce glare. Some stores are not able to scan these checks, and a manager may be called on to approve the check.

Other options are available for those who find it difficult to write standard-size checks. If someone else is filling in the checks for you to sign, but you have difficulty getting your signature to fit on the line, you can arrange with your bank to change your signature to just your first initial and last name. Another option is a check-writing guide, which is a template that is placed over a blank check. You write in the cutout slots that fit over the lines on the check. The guides are available at low vision stores.

You can avoid writing and signing checks entirely by doing what my mother and I did when she no longer could see well enough to write checks. She had me added to her checking account, and I handled all her bill paying from that point on.

CHECKS AND DEPOSITS						BALANCE
NUMBER	DATE	WRITTEN TO / RECEIVED FROM		CHECK AMOUNT	DEPOSIT AMOUNT	$
				$	$	

A large print check register

Keeping and Balancing Your Check Register

Trying to fit dollar amounts in the columns on the check registers you get from the bank is even more difficult than writing a check. You can make your own register by using a loose-leaf notebook with lined paper and columns drawn in for check number, date, payee, check amount, deposit amount, and balance. An easier solution is to buy a large print check register from a low vision store. The spaces are big enough to write in using a bold pen. Big-number and talking calculators are available to help you balance your check register.

Reducing Check Writing by Using Debit and Credit Cards

You can cut down on the number of checks you need to write for purchases by using either a bank debit card (sometimes called a check card) or a traditional credit card. With each type of card you will receive a monthly statement that itemizes the date and place of each purchase. This listing is very handy for record keeping.

When you use a debit card, the amount of your purchase is immediately deducted from your bank account. You do not have to write a check each month to cover your purchases as you do with a credit card, and this is a great convenience. However, you will be charged an overdraft fee for purchases made when you do not have sufficient funds in your account. Overdraft charges are an unnecessary expense and add up quickly, so keep a record of the amount of each purchase in your check register and don't use the card if you do not have enough money in the account to cover your purchase. Insufficient bank funds may also result in your card being denied—this is not only embarrassing, but also an annoyance if you have to leave the store without the items you wanted to purchase.

Before using a debit card, make sure you understand all the conditions of use by having someone read you the terms or by checking with the issuer of the card if the terms are difficult to interpret. Unlike issuers of credit cards, most banks will not protect you if your debit card is stolen and someone uses it to make purchases or get cash at an ATM machine. All the funds in your bank account could be wiped out, so guard your card very carefully.

With a traditional credit card, you will be sent a statement each month, and if you do not pay your balance in full you will be charged an interest fee. This expense should be avoided, as should the dangers of running up a large balance. This is not the time to incur debt, especially debt that carries a high interest rate, so consider what you are able to afford and, if possible, do not charge more than you are able to pay off each month. If you use the credit card for all your purchases, you will need to write only one check each month.

If you are a computer user, you can view a history of your transactions online, pay bills, transfer money between accounts, order checks, and perform just about any banking function while sitting in your chair at home.

Identifying Money

Finding the correct amount of money in your wallet or coin purse is another new skill that involves the sense of touch. My Uncle Matt showed me a system of keeping track of paper currency 50 years ago. It fascinated me then, and it is still in use today. It involves folding each denomination of paper money in a different way.

- One dollar: Unfolded

- Five dollars: Folded in half crosswise

- Ten dollars: Folded in quarters

- Twenty dollars: Folded in half lengthwise

If you don't like this system, develop your own or use one of these ideas.

- Put each denomination in a different pocket in your purse.

- Secure five-dollar bills with a small paper clip and ten-dollar bills with a large paper clip. Use no clips for one-dollar bills.

Coins can be identified by paying attention to their sizes and feel. It is easy to tell the difference between a quarter and a dime or penny by the coins' sizes, but what about distinguishing quarters from nickels or pennies from dimes? Quarters and dimes have ridges around their rims that you can feel with your fingernail, so it's easy to distinguish them from nickels and pennies.

To find coins quickly, you can get a wallet with four coin slots at a low vision store or you can use little coin purses for different coins—perhaps quarters and pennies in one and nickels and dimes in another.

Taking Care of Personal and Legal Affairs

"Lifetime planning" is a good way to look at the job of preparing or updating your will, establishing your health care directive (also known by other names, such as living will and health care proxy, depending on your state), and naming a power of attorney. Your decisions stated in these legal documents will ultimately affect your entire family, and it will be a gift to them to have your wishes stated in legally executed documents so that there is no question about what you want, especially in regard to health care and how your property is to be distributed.

It is not exactly a pleasant prospect to think about making these choices, but such thoughts may have been lurking in the back of your mind. If you have not yet taken any action, consider that by moving forward, you put yourself in control of deciding important issues that will arise later.

Take charge of your life by putting your wishes in legal documents and designating who you want to handle the job of carrying out those wishes. It is good to have the services of an attorney who understands the complexities of laws about property rights, taxes, wills, probate, and trusts. If the cost of hiring such an attorney is prohibitive, check with your local legal aid society or the United Way. In many areas of the United States, all you have to do is dial 211 to speak to a government human services employee who can assist you in finding such help. You may also find help from your county bar association foundation, as often members volunteer their legal services.

It is efficient and cost-effective to have all your legal documents prepared at the same time. Two witnesses are generally required for all the documents, so it is convenient to sign them all at one time.

Deciding How to Distribute Your Possessions and Writing Your Will

A will serves two purposes.

- It allows you to legally state your wishes about how you want your property to be distributed after your death.

- It designates and gives legal authority to the person or persons you want to carry out the provisions in your will.

Your property includes all your monetary assets and personal possessions, including your pets. Whether your possessions are many or few, it is important to prepare a will so that there will be no question about whom you want to receive what particular items in your estate. It is important to be very specific. Just telling a daughter or niece that you want her to have the afghan knitted by your mother does not necessarily mean she will get it. Oral promises are not legal documents, so put such gift directions in writing. Sometimes there are very surprising conflicts among relatives who all want or hoped to get the same item. It could be the turkey roaster or favorite pie pan—something with sentimental value. Painful family fights have erupted over who gets such a favorite heirloom.

Often wills state that the surviving spouse receives all the property, but you may want to give a memento or monetary gift to a child, grandchild, godchild, or friend. Receiving such a remembrance is very special for the recipient, as I learned when my Uncle Ted, who was also my godfather, named me in his will. His son, who served as his executor, sent me a check and photos my uncle had been saving all those years. I was touched beyond words. Your will is the way you can confidently make such gifts.

Naming an Executor to Handle Your Estate

You will name an executor, known as a "personal representative" in some states, whose job it will be to administer your estate. This involves locating all of the estate assets, paying its debts, expenses, and taxes, and distributing the remaining assets according to the directives of the will. Be sure to get the permission of the person or persons you wish to name as executor before designating him, her, or them in your will. And let the executor and family members know the name of your attorney.

When you ask a person to be executor of your estate, you are asking someone you trust to carry out your wishes. Even with small estates, this can be a time-consuming responsibility, and it is possible to make arrangements for compensation. The more clearly your wishes and directives are stated in your legal will, the easier you make the duties of the person you have given the honor of acting as your executor.

Saving Time and Money by Being Prepared for Meetings

Before you meet with your attorney, decide how you want your possessions distributed. Also prepare by organizing your information regarding your assets and liabilities. Provide copies of important documents, such as previous wills, trusts, power of attorney documents, life insurance policies, and employment benefits.

Preparing a Health Care Directive

You can express your preferences about the medical treatment you wish to receive at the end of your life by preparing a health care directive. With this written legal document, you ensure that:

- Your preferences will be made known, even if you are unable to express them

- The physicians will know whose direction is to be followed in the event that your family disagrees about your medical treatment

- Family members won't have to choose your care levels at what is likely one of the most stressful times of their lives

- You will have appointed an agent or agents to make decisions in accordance with your instructions about your medical care

States have differing regulations for health care directives, and some states use different names for this document. You can obtain information and forms from your state's department of health, and often from your doctor. Your attorney is perhaps the best source of information and forms. Many law firms have developed a simplified legal form, and you can have it executed at the same time that you are signing other documents. My health care directive is a legal form that was developed by my attorney's firm. I liked its provisions, so I used that form instead of the one offered by my state's department of health.

I appointed my son and my daughter as my agents, and I have discussed my wishes with them. It is good to start developing a spirit of openness with your family if you have not felt comfortable talking about end-of-life issues in the past. Or perhaps you have tried to bring up these topics and your children have changed the subject. I wish I had been more receptive when my own mother wanted to talk about what she called her "demise" and her thoughts of how things would be after that distant event. I found the topic difficult, but I now understand how much she wanted to share her thoughts and wishes and that it could have been helpful to both of us.

Authorizing Your Power of Attorney

The person you appoint as your power of attorney is commonly referred to in legal documents as "Agent" or "Attorney-in-Fact." That person is authorized to take any action on your behalf that is permitted in the document. The form is a simple one that includes a checklist of powers you want to grant, such as handling real property or acting for you if you become incapacitated or incompetent. I have again designated my son and my daughter as my powers of attorney.

Power of attorney documents should be drawn up by your lawyer, paralegal, or estate representative. Your goal is to assign a person or persons power of attorney in all matters, with all organizations, as defined in your document. Some institutions, such as banks, may offer to draw up a power of attorney agreement that will allow your agent access to your bank funds and that will authorize him or her to write checks against your accounts.

However, such an agreement has no legal bearing on any other institution, such as utility companies, credit card companies, hospitals, the IRS, and other organizations that your agent might need to deal with on your behalf. Without the proper, state-authorized power of attorney in place, your agent may find himself or herself unable even to get the information needed to pay a bill or settle your taxes in a timely manner.

Many people do not realize that power of attorney is void immediately upon the death of the person who has given that power of attorney. At that point, bank accounts and other assets may be frozen until the estate goes through probate. This is one good reason for your agent to have additional access to funds to handle outstanding bills and funeral expenses. There are several ways to handle this. One is to have your agent signed onto your bank account so that he or she can write checks from the account even after your death. You can also have your credit card company add your agent as a co-user of the card, with equal responsibility for payments owed. My son and I "share" a credit card, in part because he is very kind about doing shopping errands for me, but also so that he will be able to use the card to pay my final expenses. If you would rather not add your executor or power of attorney to your bank accounts or credit cards, you might just provide your executor funds, in the form of cash, ahead of time so that he or she has the money to handle funeral and other expenses.

Keeping Your Documents Safe and Accessible

It's a good idea to store most of the originals of all valuable documents in a safe-deposit box, and to keep copies in your home.

A large vault inside a bank is the most common location for safe-deposit boxes. To rent a box, you and the others you want to have access must sign a lease agreement. Two acceptable forms of identification are generally required. It is a time-consuming matter to add or remove someone's name, so allow time if that becomes necessary. Think ahead about whom you want to have access to your box, because it is where you will keep your valuables and important documents.

- Understand that, in most cases, your designated power of attorney has access to the box any time up to your death, not just in the event of your illness. However, upon your death that power of attorney is voided, and no one other than those you have previously arranged to have access may get to your safe-deposit box and its contents for some time. Unfortunately, some important documents that may be kept in the box might be needed immediately. For this reason, consider setting up your safe-deposit account with at least one other person, who will have unlimited access to the box (and who will assume responsibility for it after your death).

- You will probably get two keys. Keep one in a safe place and give the other to another signer on the box. Let each other know where you keep the key.

- The keys you receive when you lease your box are the only keys that will open the box. If you lose a key, report it to the bank immediately. You will probably incur a charge for this. If both keys are lost you will probably have to pay a locksmith to open the box and replace the lock.

- Pay your rental fees on time—if you don't, any property in the box might be turned over to your state's unclaimed property office. It is handy to have the fees automatically deducted from your account on a monthly or annual basis.

- Do not use the safe-deposit box to store documents you might need when the bank is closed, such as power-of-attorney papers or, possibly, the original of your health care directive.

In addition to keeping documents in a safe-deposit box, you will probably want to have copies—and, in some cases, the originals—in your home. Some hospitals will not honor photocopies of health care directives, particularly if the hospital staff takes issue with any stipulations made in those directives. Note that most paramedics are trained to look for health care directives posted on the refrigerator when they come to a person's home. For these reasons, you may want to keep the original of your health care directive there—in plain view, in a sealed plastic bag, to prevent it from becoming stained or damaged—with copies in your safe-deposit box, in the possession of your power of attorney, and with your spouse and children.

Preplanning Funerals

Some people like to plan everything ahead—even their own funerals. Others don't want to think about such an idea. I helped a friend from high school who had heart failure plan her funeral, down to the details of selecting the paper for the programs and choosing the music from selections performed by a musician friend at her bedside. My longtime friend and I actually had fun working out all the details, and it gave her great comfort to plan the service. On the other hand, my husband did not want to hear anything about the plans we were making and said he thought the whole thing was bizarre.

If you want to preplan your arrangements, note that there are formal ways to do so.

- Many houses of worship can help you plan ahead. I attended a workshop at my church and received a form to note my choices for music and readings. The information will be entered in a database.

- Funeral homes have preplanning guides in which you can enter your choices for everything from flowers to type of burial. In addition to preplanning your service, you can prepay for your funeral through the funeral home you select. This is another way to gain peace of mind and to relieve your family of a difficult task.

Although such decisions are difficult to contemplate, making your wishes known can give you peace of mind and can help your family by removing their burden of having to make decisions under the most adverse conditions.

─── MY STORY ───

One Day Too Late for My Husband

When my husband and I last saw our family attorney, who was about to retire, our wills were six years old. He advised us to update them, as they were at that point irrelevant because our children were grown. I just stuck the name of the new attorney he recommended in a file folder. Year after year went by until 10 more years had passed. The wills were now 16 years old, and my husband was less and less inclined to discuss such a topic. In our marriage, I handled all the bill paying, taxes, appointments, and legal affairs, so it was up to me to follow through and contact the new attorney. My rationale for procrastinating was that broaching the subject would be too upsetting for my husband.

Then his health began to fail and he started kidney dialysis. He became more and more fearful, and I was more scared than ever to bring up subjects such as wills, health directives, and cemetery plots. I finally got up the courage to tell my husband I wanted to talk to him about our wills. The existing documents were so out of date that they even listed a guardian for our children, who were all now well beyond childhood. My husband seemed almost relieved to be having the discussion, and he told me to go ahead and call the attorney to prepare wills that would include the changes we decided to make.

Again I procrastinated. A month passed, and in February my husband was rushed to the emergency room and later released to a nursing home. I still did not call the attorney. In March I made the call and learned we needed entirely new wills, along with health care directives and powers of attorney. My husband was growing weaker, so I told him about the attorney's sample health care directive and its provisions about care in the event of a coma. He said to go ahead with that document and, although this wasn't covered in the health care directive, he told me his wishes regarding resuscitation. I think we both felt a sense of relief for having confronted these issues.

After that the attorney and I worked quickly. My husband and I had almost duplicate documents, but it took some weeks to work out all the details. My husband had decided that he would like to give special gifts of cash to our son and daughter, and these gifts were listed in the will in heartfelt language. We made a date for signing the documents on April 18, and I arranged to have a room for our meeting at the nursing home. But on April 17 he was rushed back to the hospital. I called the attorney to postpone our meeting. Things did not seem that serious, but two days later my husband had sudden complications and was rushed to intensive care. The family and six doctors and nurses surrounded his bed, and the lead doctor presented three care options. Our family knew exactly what he wanted and immediately told the doctors. They started to thank us, and I couldn't understand why. I took a doctor aside and asked, and he said it was rare for a family to immediately know the patient's wishes and to all agree on carrying them out. Often the doctors are confronted with quarreling family members and care is delayed while they try to reach an agreement. Our knowing what to do was a blessing not only to us, but also to the doctors. And to my husband. He died on April 19. He did not see or have the chance to sign the will and the other documents.

My procrastination meant that we had no cemetery plots. At the workshop I'd heard about something new to me— renting a casket for the visitation and service, followed by cremation and placement of the urn in a mausoleum. On the way to the funeral home to make arrangements, I told my children about this possibility and that I liked the idea. So did they, and as I had no hint of what my husband would want, other than being with me, we decided on the rental casket/cremation plan. Our decision was made in the space of five minutes in a car when we were under extreme and painful stress. It was not a good place or time to decide something so important.

A few weeks after my husband's death my daughter was back in town, so it was time to tell her and my son about their gifts. Although I wasn't legally required to do so because our new wills had not been finalized, I wanted to carry out my husband's wishes, and I was able to fund their gifts from our joint assets. After a nice dinner at home, I told them that their father had left them special gifts, and I read his words from the draft of his will. They were surprised and moved beyond words. My deep regret is that I was unable to show them an executed will, with their father's signature at the end.

9

Embracing Technology

OPEN YOUR MIND to the ways in which technology can keep you connected to your world. Do not allow yourself to become detached from your everyday life, but rather use the adaptive digital products described in this chapter to find new ways to maintain your current contacts and interests. In this chapter, three categories of products are described.

- Audio technology, which enables you to "listen" to books and magazines that are read aloud
- Video magnifiers, which display enlarged images of print and photos on a screen
- Computers and related technology, which enable you to prepare documents, connect to the Internet, and use e-mail

Audio Technology:
Listening to Talking Books

The lives of people with vision loss have been enriched over the last 75 years by listening to recordings of books and magazines from the Talking Book Program of the National Library Service for the Blind and Physically Handicapped (NLS), which is administered by the Library of Congress. The NLS is a free program that loans recorded and braille books and magazines in a number of languages, music scores in braille and in large print, and specially designed playback equipment to U.S. residents and American citizens domiciled abroad. There is no minimum age requirement. Enrollment is open to those who are unable to read or use standard print materials because of visual or physical impairment. The ease of listening to recorded material has steadily improved over the years thanks to the adoption of new technology—most recently digital audio.

Origins of the NLS and Its Talking Book Program

The history of Talking Books and the NLS illustrates how the latest technology can be applied to continually make things in our lives more and more accessible. The NLS was established by the Pratt-Smoot Act in 1931, which provided funds to establish a national library program to provide books for blind adult readers. The service is administered by the Library of Congress. The slogan of the NLS is "That All May Read," and anyone who has an inability to see or hold standard printed materials is eligible to receive books and magazines through the program.

Development of Talking Books and Their Machines

Seventy-five years ago, when the first recordings were made available, the format used was the 33⅓ rpm, 12-inch disc, which was played on a special machine. During the next 25 years the machines were improved, with many refinements made to their motors and operating features. By 1963 all books were recorded at 16⅔ rpm. Audiocassette tapes were first used for recording in 1969, and the analog cassette book and cassette book machine technology were the backbone of the system for 30 years. New models of playback machines were developed over the years, and in 1990 the first talking book machine with variable speed control was produced. This analog system became obsolete by the early 2000s, and the move to digital technology began.

For a detailed chronology of the Talking Book Program, visit the NLS Web site (www.loc.gov/nls/about_history.html).

The Move to Digital Technology

In 2008 the Talking Book Program started the transition to a new digital flash memory system. This system uses a cartridge with a special playback machine that is much smaller and lighter than the cassette player, making the equipment easier to use. There will be a long transition period during which the program will continue to provide cassettes and their players, but ultimately digital formats will replace audiocassette technology, just as audiocassette technology replaced its predecessor, the rigid disc. The move to digital technology is expected to be completed by 2012.

The flash cartridge system offers several advantages over the cassette system.

- Smaller size—the digital player measures about 6 by 9 by 2 inches, compared to the cassette player's 9 by 11 by 3 inches

- Lighter weight—the digital player is slightly over two pounds, compared to seven pounds for the cassette player

- Improved audio reproduction, which provides better audio quality for listeners

- Larger storage capacities—one cartridge can contain an entire book, compared to multiple cassettes for each book

- Elimination of the need to turn the cassette over and flip a switch to access the other side

- Easier portability of recordings and machines

- Less storage space required for collections at network libraries

- Long life of cartridges and the ability to replay a cartridge many times while retaining high-quality audio output

- Relatively simple duplication process for libraries to produce copies on cartridges

- Widely available, mature technology with rapidly declining prices

The second phase of the move to digital technology is the digital download project, by which patrons can download material from the Internet. The third stage is focused on cartridge duplication on demand, whereby digital titles are produced when requested by users. Cartridges are recycled during this process, making it a very cost-efficient mode.

Enrolling in the Talking Books Program

United States residents and citizens living abroad who meet one of the following criteria are eligible to participate in the Talking Book Program.

- Persons whose visual disability, with correction and regardless of optical measurement, is certified by competent authority as preventing the reading of standard printed material

- Persons certified by competent authority as unable to read or unable to use standard printed material as a result of physical limitations
- Persons certified by competent authority as having a reading disability

Note that the official eligibility criteria include certification of one's eligibility by a "competent authority." Per its Web site, the NLS defines "competent authority" to include:

- Doctors of medicine, doctors of osteopathy, ophthalmologists, and optometrists
- Registered nurses, therapists, and professional staff of hospitals and institutions
- Public or private welfare agency employees, including social workers, caseworkers, counselors, rehabilitation teachers, and superintendents

In the absence of any of these, certification may be made by a professional librarian or by any person whose competence under specific circumstances is acceptable to the Library of Congress.

How the Program Works

Once you are enrolled, you will receive a playback machine from the regional center that provides the players. During the technological transition period, the new digital cartridge players may be in short supply in your state, so it is possible that you will receive a cassette player instead of a cartridge player. (The cassette and cartridge systems will run as dual programs until the conversion to the cartridge system is complete.)

When you are enrolled, you will start receiving the free publication *Talking Book Topics*, which is published every two months and is available in large print, on audiocassette, and on the NLS Web site. The annotated list in each issue is limited to titles recently added to the national collection, which contains thousands of fiction and nonfiction titles including classics, biographies, Gothics, mysteries, and how-to and self-help guides. There are special sections for children's and foreign language books. To learn more about the books in the national collection, readers can order catalogs and bibliographies by subject from cooperating libraries. Librarians can check other resources for titles and answer requests about special materials.

To order audio recordings of books and magazines, check with your regional library for its options. All material is delivered directly to you free by U.S. mail, and you return it, at no postage cost, to the library. This door-to-door delivery service is an extremely valuable part of the program.

--- **MY STORY** ---

From Reading with Uncle Matt to Downloading Books

When my Uncle Matt lost his central vision over 50 years ago, he was a practicing tax attorney who lived in St. Paul,

Minnesota. He took the streetcar, by himself with his white cane, to the neighboring city of Minneapolis to learn braille at what was then called the Minneapolis Society for the Blind, but which now is known as Vision Loss Resources. After class he sometimes took the streetcar to our house in Minneapolis, where he would spread out his large braille sheets on the dining room table and proudly demonstrate how he could read. Before long he became a volunteer lawyer at a legal aid society.

Uncle Matt's hobby and great interest was the Civil War, and he missed being able to read new books on the subject as they were published. Back then there were a few Talking Book recordings on 33⅓ rpm records, but the program didn't offer recorded books on relatively specialized topics such as the Civil War. If he lived today, he would find 1,458 entries for the Civil War in the online catalog of the National Library Service holdings. To help fill the Civil War void in my uncle's life, my husband-to-be and I made weekly trips to his house, where we took turns reading aloud the new books he could no longer see.

Thirty years later my mother, then in her late 70s, learned she had macular degeneration after the cataract surgery she'd expected to restore her vision made no improvement. Always an avid reader, her life began to revolve around Talking Books. I visited her every Wednesday, and the main activity was me reading aloud the list of new books available and writing down the order for her selections. I kept a log of these selections in a notebook that I still have. Her cassette playback machine was awkward, the sound was poor, and she had to pass over many books she wanted to hear because she couldn't understand many high-pitched female voices. It was difficult for her, while listening to a book, to keep track of the many cassette tapes that were required for most books. Still, with her life enhanced by her beloved Talking Books, my mother went on to live a life of spirited acceptance until she died at the age of 88.

Now, 20 years later, I look forward to the day when I can catch up on all the reading I have never been able to fit into my life. But I will not be waiting for a visitor to read to me or struggling with cassettes and their playback machine. Instead I will be listening to books on a lightweight cartridge machine or, more likely, downloading books from the Talking Book Internet site. This is an exciting and comforting prospect for me.

Video Magnifiers: Start by Using Simple Devices

Simplicity is the goal as you use technology to connect to your world. If a simple aid, such as an ordinary magnifying glass described in chapter 3, provides you the help you need, do not complicate your life by using advanced products that your current level of vision does not yet require. You may have years before you need any special help, and then you can gradually start using more complex aids as you need them. The goal is to be open to the assistive technology that is there to help people with varying levels of vision loss and to know the types of products that are available.

Enlarging with Video Magnifiers (CCTVs)

Video magnifiers are often called closed-circuit televisions (CCTVs) because they use a camera to take a photo of the material to be viewed and show a magnified image of that material on a screen. CCTV technology allows for greater magnification than does a magnifying glass. There is, however, a sharp difference in the cost of a video magnifier and a simple magnifying glass, with low-end video magnifiers costing well over a hundred dollars and high-end magnifiers costing thousands of dollars. Both stationary desktop and portable models are available. Variable levels of magnification are available within each unit, depending on the particular model. Some models show images in color—these are great for looking at photos.

Handheld Portable Video Magnifiers with Built-In Screens (CCTVs)

Handheld magnifiers are made up of a camera and a built-in screen in the four- to six-inch size range. In product catalogs, these devices are frequently listed in the video magnifier category. The magnifiers are placed over the material to be viewed and the image is displayed on the screen. You can bring these portable magnifiers with you to read print material when you are out and about. They are lightweight and fit easily into pockets and purses. They are useful for:

- Reading price tags on clothing items or food labels at the grocery store
- Magnifying and illuminating menus at restaurants

Desktop Video Magnifiers (CCTVs)

This type of magnifier looks like a computer because it has a monitor that is similar to a computer screen. In product catalogs, desktop video magnifiers are generally called CCTVs, or sometimes reading systems. You place your material on a viewing table that you move to position your material under the stationary video camera above the table. A magnified image of the text or photos is displayed on the screen. You move the material by sliding the table side-to-side and up and down. Screens are available in various sizes, and you can adjust the size of the magnification to meet your visual needs. Desktop magnifiers are useful for:

- Reading documents, books, and newspapers
- Viewing photos
- Writing checks

- Recording deposits and withdrawals in your check register

Handheld Video Magnifiers (CCTVs) that Plug into TVs or Computers

With this type of video magnifier, you use your own TV or computer monitor to display images, so the cost of a handheld video magnifier is much less than that of a desktop model. The device, which is sometimes called a mouse magnifier because of the shape of one model, is actually a small handheld camera. To operate it, you plug the cord of the device into the USB port of your computer or into your television set. You place the material you want to display on a table or desk, and move the device over the material. The camera then scans the material and displays it on the screen, in the magnification you have chosen from the options available with your brand and model. Handheld video magnifiers are useful for:

- Reading documents, books, and newspapers
- Viewing photos

Reading with Scanner Readers That Convert Text to Speech

Unlike magnifiers that display images on a screen, scanner readers convert written material into spoken words by using OCR (optical character recognition) technology after a printed document is scanned by a camera. To operate this device, you hold the reader over printed material and push a button to snap a picture of the material. Next, OCR software converts the scanned image into recognized characters and words. Finally, a synthesizer speaks the recognized text. Scanner readers can:

- Read most printed material, including letters, bills, receipts, ATM slips, business cards, text documents, and office memos

- Read items such as restaurant menus and airline boarding passes (portable units only)

- Save captured images for future playback or delete them immediately—thousands of printed pages can be stored by adding extra memory, and users can transfer files to their desktops and laptop computers

Portable Multifunction Scanner Readers/Magnifiers

This multifunction category includes a handheld portable reading machine that also has magnification and multimedia access to audio books and music. The device has a camera at the rear of the unit, a 7-inch video screen, and two controls—one for each thumb—to navigate through various functions, including:

- Reading restaurant menus, newspapers, magazines, and product labels

- Enlarging the image of any item
- Listening to music or books stored on the device

Computer Technology for Writing, Reading, Speaking, and Hearing

If you are not already using a computer, consider getting started. Computers can open up new worlds to you, from keeping in touch with children and grandchildren by e-mail to accessing the Internet and finding information on any topic. If you are nervous about your ability to successfully navigate in the world of computers and related technology, consider that many people with age-related diseases have had their first successful experiences with computers only after their vision loss. There are endless adaptive strategies for using a computer, ranging from special keyboards with large, contrasting letters to software programs that read aloud the text that is displayed on the monitor.

Refresh Typing Skills and Get a Large-Letter Keyboard

If it has been several years since you used a typewriter or a keyboard, you can update your skills by practicing touch typing and training your fingers to know the location of each key. If you have difficulty seeing the letters on the keyboard, you can get a keyboard with large, bold letters. Large-letter keyboards are available with black letters on white, black letters on yellow, and white letters on black. The hunt-and-peck system may work for you for a while, but you will be better served by learning touch typing. Classes are available in community education programs, senior centers, and other locations. SeniorNet is a very useful organization that offers both online and classroom courses in locations throughout the country. See page 201 for more information.

Selecting a Computer and Monitor

If you do not already own a computer, check with family members and friends before you purchase one, as someone may have an older model that he or she would be happy to give you. The more important component is actually the monitor. Use a digital, flat-screen monitor for sharp resolution and ease in reading. Look for a model with a screen that can tilt backward and forward, as one of those

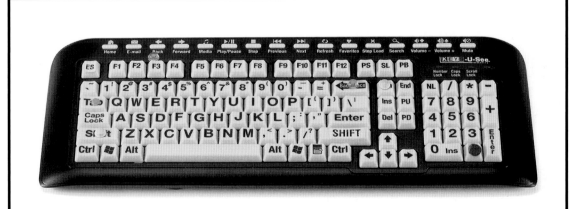

A keyboard with bold black letters on yellow keys

positions may make it easier for you to view the text or images that are on the screen. Get a model that has buttons on the front to change the brightness and contrast levels. You will find that different programs vary in their brightness, so you can suddenly be faced with glare when you switch to a new application. You want to be able to lower the brightness level with a quick push of a button to ease the discomfort of glare. Just remember: if you go to another application and you find that the toolbars are so dark you cannot read menus or distinguish icons, switch to a new level of brightness.

Using Computers' Standard Accessibility Options

Computers come with preinstalled options that help people with low vision see what is on the screen. PC and Macintosh (Mac) computers come with different assistive options; highlights of each system are given below. If you have not used a computer before, you might want to bring this book to a computer store and have a sales associate show you, on an actual computer, the various features discussed here.

Windows Operating Systems on PC Computers

Windows has an accessibility wizard that allows you to select different features to help you see what is on the monitor. Here are some of the settings you can change.

- Scroll bar size

- Window border size

- Desktop icon size

- Desktop color and contrast

- Cursor size and blink rate

Microsoft Office programs allow you to enlarge the size and font of the type that appears on the screen. Adobe Reader has a Text-to-Speech (TTS) tool, called "Read Out Loud," that can read aloud a single page or an entire PDF document.

Macintosh Operating Systems on Apple Computers

Apple's Macintosh (Mac) computers contain several technologies to assist you in seeing and hearing what is on the computer screen. These technologies are part of the computer's operating system and do not require special software. Any text can be read aloud within every program except iPhotos. You can also hear a description of what is on your screen. Other useful accessibility features include:

- Zoom options that allow for magnification of up to 40 times, with a preview rectangle that outlines the portion of the screen that will be magnified

- Display adjustment options that allow text to appear as white on black

- Contrast adjustment, for varying degrees of contrast

- Scalable cursor options that allow you to make the cursor appear larger on the screen so that it is easier to find and follow when you move the mouse

Speech recognition is also available in the Macintosh Leopard operating system, but only for computer commands. You would need to purchase a separate software program to have your own spoken words appear on the screen.

Advancing to Special Accessibility Software

There is special software for computers that goes far beyond the features that come automatically with the operating systems. One category is speech recognition software; another is screen-reading software. The difference between the two applications can be confusing. The distinction is that, with speech recognition software, you do the talking into a microphone and your words appear on the screen as text, and with screen-reading software, the computer talks to you through a speech synthesizer and reads aloud what is on the screen.

Speech Recognition Software

Speech recognition software is available for both PC and Macintosh computers. After a short training session in which you read a list of words that teaches the software to recognize your voice patterns, you speak into a microphone and your words and sentences appear on the screen. You do not need to see or use the keyboard. For this reason, speech recognition software is especially useful for people with very poor vision and for poor typists.

With speech recognition software you can prepare any kind of document and write e-mail messages. With each new version of software, the accuracy rate increases, but it is a good idea to have what appears on the screen checked for missing letters and incorrect punctuation.

Screen-Reading Software That Requires Typing

Screen-reading software is available for PC computers. It works by recognizing and speaking aloud the information displayed on the computer screen using synthesized speech through your computer's sound card. A selection of male and female voices is available to do the reading. Some screen-reading software programs also magnify the computer screen to fit your level of vision. Use this category of software for:

- Creating and editing Microsoft Office documents by typing and using simple commands

- Hearing a spoken echo of each key or word as you type; you can choose to have all keys or only selected groups of keys "spoken" as they are struck

- Reading aloud of documents and e-mail by the speech synthesizer

- Accessing the Internet and the reading aloud of any Web page

Internet-Access Software with No Typing Required

Another category of software enables you to access the Internet and receive and send e-mail without typing. These programs read aloud what is on the screen, in the voice you have chosen from a selection of male and female voices. You can also read the screen in a choice of magnifications to fit your visual needs. It is easy to learn how to use these programs; they require very little training.

When you start the program, the software's synthesized voice tells you options that you can select, such as e-mail or reading the newspaper on the Internet. You pick which option you want by:

- Clicking the mouse when you hear that option
- Choosing to have new e-mail messages read to you or displayed on the screen
- Sending a message by either speaking into a microphone attached to your computer or by typing the message

An important feature is the way in which the software organizes information. This is done in a number of useful ways, including:

- Listing certain sites you can go to directly without navigating the broader Internet

- Presenting what is available on the Internet in an organized group of broad categories such as news, weather, and entertainment

- Listing specific groupings within these broad categories—for example, under the news category there are subcategories such as business, finance, and local news by state

Obtaining Technological Products

Most of the products that are described in this chapter are available from one or more of the low vision stores listed in Appendix A. In Appendix B, a list of representative manufacturers and U.S. distributors is presented. By visiting manufacturers' Web sites, getting information over the phone, and visiting stores that sell these items, you can learn about the latest products in the ever-changing field of assistive technology.

The products mentioned in this chapter, unlike those discussed in other chapters, can cost hundreds and even thousands of dollars. If costs are prohibitive, you may be able to get one or more of these products free, at a reduced cost, or on loan through one of several organizations. Some of these organizations are listed below and are described fully in chapter 11. You will need to meet financial and visual-impairment criteria, and you may be put on a waiting list because the products are often in short supply.

Each state has a Commissioner for the Blind that operates services for the blind and visually handicapped. See page 206 for information on how to find the agency in your state. Agencies usually have products on display, and home visits may be made by counselors to assess your situation and determine whether or not you qualify for state services. Equipment that is given or loaned to you will be brought to your home, and you will receive instruction on how to use each device.

Lions Clubs in some communities also offer assistance. And if you are a veteran, you might want to consult the Department of Veterans Affairs, which has several programs that offer both equipment and training.

Forge Ahead into the World of Technology

Think of technological products as your assistants in helping you to operate in a world of diminished vision. From the array of product types described in this chapter, explore and adopt the ones that are right for you. Do not be scared off by thinking they will be difficult to use—as you will learn in the next chapter, there are people and organizations that are ready to help you. And if you are not already a computer user, you can give yourself a head start by developing computer skills right now.

PART 4

Maximizing Your Independence

YOUR STRATEGIC PLAN for living well with vision loss includes an important goal—maintaining as much independence as you are safely able to do. In earlier chapters you learned practical ideas for doing everyday things in new ways. This section turns to keeping control over important areas of your life—driving and maximizing independence through the selective assistance of others. Chapter 10 discusses making decisions about driving. Chapter 11 describes the many resources available to help you stay as independent as possible—once you decide you are ready to seek assistance from people and organizations. This can be a difficult adjustment to make. Needing others can make you feel powerless, but consider that it is you who can choose if and when to seek that help.

10

Making Driving Decisions

DRIVING SAFELY involves many factors, and good vision is only one of them. Strength and agility are also needed because driving involves the use of most of the muscle groups in the body, as explained on pages 44–45. Although the loss of ability to drive safely is one of the most difficult things to face, it may help to remember that even people with excellent vision may be forced to stop driving if they lack the health or motor skills required to safely operate an automobile.

Should I Still Be Driving?

Safety—for you, your passengers, people in other vehicles, bikers, and pedestrians—must be the prime consideration when you decide whether or not it is still all right for you to drive. Even if you still have a valid driver's license, you may decide that it is time to stop driving.

If you can be honest with yourself, you will be the best judge of if, when, and where you should be driving. Ask yourself these questions.

- Do I feel unsafe when I'm driving, even on familiar routes?
- Do vehicles or people seem to appear suddenly out of nowhere?
- Do I have physical issues, such as slow reaction time or inability to turn my head or my upper body, that hinder my ability to check for other vehicles?
- Are other people reluctant to get in the car with me when I'm the driver?
- Have family members or friends suggested it's time I stop driving?
- Do I become panicky or lose confidence when I find myself in congested or fast-moving traffic?

If your answer to any of these questions is yes, it is time for you to figure out if it is time for you to stop driving. To help you decide, professional assessments are offered by occupational therapists and some rehabilitation centers. You take charge of deciding how to making the decision.

I'm Driving for Now

If you are still driving, consider adopting self-imposed restrictions such as not driving at night or when it is raining or snowing, staying within a comfortable speed limit, traveling only on local roads with which you are familiar, and canceling trips if the weather is threatening.

Renewing Your Driver's License—the Vision Test

When the time to renew your driver's license approaches, you may find it helpful to prepare for the vision test by following these tips. States vary in their minimum vision requirements for passing the test, so cutoff points are not listed here.

■ Plan to take the test a few weeks ahead of your birthday—don't wait until the last minute, when you will be more anxious about passing because of the deadline.

■ Take the test on a day when both you and your eyes are feeling especially good—a day when you feel confident.

■ Get someone to drive you to the test so you don't become nervous just getting to the licensing bureau.

■ Ask that your driver come in with you, as you might need help in filling out the renewal application form. When I recently applied, my son had to fill out the form because it was so dark at the writing table that I could not read the questions or write the answers.

■ If you do not pass the test, you may be eligible for a restricted license if it is offered in your state. Besides wearing eyeglasses, restrictions can include no nighttime driving, no freeway driving, no driving beyond limited areas or routes, and no driving above a certain speed. Some states require a recommendation on restrictions from an eye doctor; others may determine restrictions at the licensing bureau.

Take a Driver Safety Class

These classes are offered by many different organizations and are called by various names, including "Driver Safety Program" (AARP), "Senior Driver Improvement Classes" (AAA), and "Defensive Driving Class." They are offered at community centers, senior centers, churches, and many other types of locations. The basic course is an eight-hour session that is usually offered in two four-hour segments, although sometimes an all-day course is offered on the weekend. In most states, insurance rates are discounted for those who have taken such courses. Refresher courses, which generally consist of one four-hour session, can be taken as often as you wish, but to retain insurance discounts, the refresher course is generally required every three years. The price of the courses runs in the $10-to-$20 range.

In the class, you can expect to learn about current rules of the road, how to operate your vehicle more safely, and how to make some adjustments to common age-related changes in vision, hearing, and reaction time. Here is a list of some of the specific topics that may be covered.

Maintaining the proper distance from other moving vehicles

Changing lanes and making turns at intersections in the safest ways

Knowing the effects of medications on driving ability

Minimizing the effects of dangerous blind spots

Eliminating driver distractions such as eating, smoking, and cell phone use

Properly using safety belts, air bags, and antilock brakes

Continuing to monitor your own and others' driving skills and capabilities

Online courses are now available in many states through AARP and other organizations but, at least for the first course, it is recommended that you attend a class in person. The give-and-take of class discussions alone is worth making the trip to the classroom.

Preparing Yourself and Your Car

Before you start off on your drive, it is very important to prepare for the trip, even if it's a short trip to a familiar place. Use the checklist below to ensure that you are prepared before you get behind the wheel.

Make sure you have the proper glasses for driving. If you have separate reading and distance glasses, get an extra pair of distance glasses to keep permanently in the car, and always store them in a dedicated location.

- Keep a pair of tinted NoIR sunglasses, described on pages 19–20, in a dedicated location in the car.

- Practice this trick for times when the sun is periodically blocked by clouds or when the sun is not bright at the start of a trip and wearing sunglasses would make the road look too dark, but sunny weather is expected during your drive. Keep your sunglasses handy by putting them above your regular glasses, and just slide them down when you're confronted with glare. Push them back up off your driving glasses when the sunlight has diminished.

- Assess the weather and check weather forecasts. If rain or snow is falling or is predicted, consider postponing the trip, as you do not want to be stranded and unable to drive back home. If it is a sunny day and you are

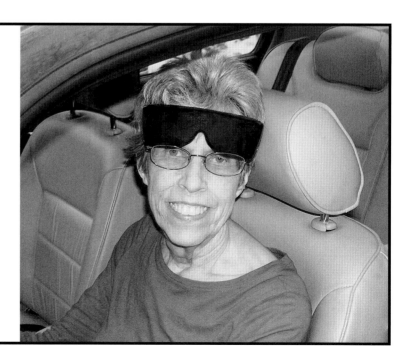

Sunglasses perched on top of driving glasses

sensitive to glare even when wearing sunglasses, consider postponing your trip or finding another means of transportation.

- Put raised bumps on dashboard buttons, such as those for the heater and defroster, so you can quickly locate them by feel. Practice reaching for the bumps before you drive to see if you are able to quickly find them.

- Check your seat position and mirrors, and make adjustments if necessary.

- Make speedometer readings visible if your dashboard is too dark for you to see the numbers by putting big white dots made with typewriter correction fluid at the numbers for 20, 40, and 60 miles per hour.

- Show fuel levels by putting a white dot at the half-full or quarter-full level.

Big white dots at 20, 40, and 60 help you to monitor your speed

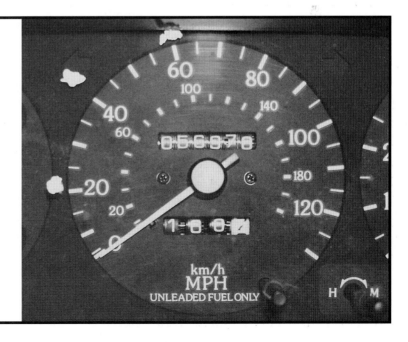

Driving the Car

The following driving pointers can help keep you safe on the road.

Stay alert at all times.

Do what you need to do to feel safe.

Concentrate on the cars ahead, but glance periodically at the side and rear mirrors.

Know your weak spots, such as slow reaction time or the need for lots of light, and drive accordingly.

Stay fit and flexible—all parts of the body are involved in driving.

If you encounter glare from an oncoming car's headlights, avert your eyes and look straight ahead.

Plan to be home before dark. Check the time of sunset, estimate how long you'll be gone, add a half hour for delays, and then work backward to figure out when you must begin to drive home in order to get back before dusk.

—————————— **MY STORY** ——————————

Taxi Al and Other Drivers

Two weeks after passing the vision test for my driver's license renewal, I noticed a loss of vision in my right eye; that experience is recounted on pages 16–18. I had already become more careful about where I'd drive, but after learning there was bleeding in my eye and receiving an injection as treatment, I had to reassess my ability to drive at all. A couple of weeks earlier I had called a taxicab company when I needed a ride to a doctor's appointment that would have required me to drive on an unfamiliar freeway. I immediately liked the driver who answered the call, so I asked if he could pick me up after the appointment and if I could arrange rides ahead of time. He responded by handing me a card that read, "TAXI-AL at your service." I discovered that he lived close by me and would schedule trips far in advance if I called him directly. Two days after my eye injection he took me to my volunteer job. I now schedule trips to the doctor and other places with him weeks in advance. We have become good friends, and it is a comfort to have him waiting for me after a difficult medical procedure.

Then there is my longstanding arrangement with my friend Arlys. We have held season orchestra tickets for 15 years, and for the last six she has been the driver because I no longer can drive at night. I'm not far out of her way, but it is still a detour. To show my appreciation, I pay for the parking. She is happy with the arrangement, and our bonus is that all those hours spent together in the car have firmly cemented our friendship.

There are other drivers in my life that I can call on occasionally, and one came from an unexpected source. Reiko, my ballet teacher, knew I'd missed a class because of threatening rain—I will not take the chance of being stranded because of a rainstorm—and she asked a young student, Amy, who lives near me to start taking me to and from a summer class, which was held some distance from my home. Because Reiko had made this arrangement without consulting me, I was upset and not the least bit gracious—in fact, I called her a mother hen. Amy insisted it would be her pleasure to drive me there and back, but I found that hard to believe. It was difficult to admit to myself that I should no longer make that drive to class, but it was even harder to receive unsolicited help. This was a new role for me, and it is one that I am still learning to accept. It has helped that Amy and I enjoy our time together and that we have become fast friends during our trips.

My most important driver is my son. He comes to work in our home office every weekday and, although we have agreed that I will not ask him to use his work time to drive me long distances, he does run short errands for me and he takes me to my regular appointments with my retinologist, whose office is nearby. I do not feel reluctant to ask my children to drive me to important places such as a doctor's office, and I have great gratitude that they so willingly help me in this way.

"Later" Has Arrived— Giving Up the Keys

Giving up driving is actually a gradual process. Long before you make the decision not to drive at all, you will probably have had to cancel a trip or find a ride when the weather or other factors prevented you from driving. But the "final" day is one that is long dreaded. **You** be the one to make the reasonable decision of when that day has arrived. This will preserve your dignity and prevent a "taking away the keys" scene with your children or friends.

These ideas may make it easier to give up the keys.

- Add up the cost of gasoline, car repairs, and automobile insurance for the previous year. That is the amount that you now have to spend on taxicabs each year, with no additional expense to your overall budget.

- Make these savings a special fund. Use a "taxi jar" for ready cash or set up a special checking account where you deposit the amount of your former car insurance or car payments on their old due dates.

- If you sell your car, realize that those proceeds are a one-time windfall. Rather than adding the amount to the taxi jar, consider putting it in a "fun fund" for trips for yourself—not for doctor's appointments or other trips made out of necessity.

- Find a taxi driver you like, ask for his or her card, and call directly when you need a ride.

- Look for a private driver—you might find one whose services are less expensive than the cost of multiple taxi trips.

- Ask for rides from relatives and friends, and think of favors to do in return, such as paying for parking, buying a few gallons of gas or a fun gift, or treating them to dinner at a nice restaurant.

- Use the transportation services that are available in almost every community or county through aging or disability services as mandated by the Americans with Disabilities Act of 1990. See pages 182–183 for more information. You will probably need to go through an application process to become eligible for these services. The services usually provide door-to-door pickup and delivery back home, and the cost per trip is very reasonable.

- Check with Medicaid, if you are in the program, to see if costs of transportation services to get you to medical appointments are covered.

- If your community has a good public transit system, you have yet another alternative for transportation.

Now relax and enjoy your trips as a passenger. Be grateful that there will be no more of those expeditions that turn terrifying when it starts to rain or you get lost trying to go somewhere new. Relish the peace of mind that both you and your loved ones will have knowing that you are safe when on the road.

11

Getting Help from People and Organizations

OPEN YOUR HEART and your mind to the prospect of reaping great rewards by accepting help from other people—your friends, family, doctors and other medical specialists—and the professional staff in organizations that are there to assist you. You can sustain and even expand the horizons of your life by utilizing the myriad opportunities available to people with vision loss. Be proactive and use the information in this chapter to find just the type of assistance you want at any particular time. Calling on others can be a difficult adjustment because it can make you feel powerless, but you are in control of deciding if, when, and where you choose to seek help. Share your feelings with family and friends. Let them know that there will be times when you need to call on them for help, but that you are in charge of your own life and are exploring the resources available in your community, as well as on a national level. This chapter tells you about different kinds of help that is available and offers a list of national organizations that are particularly suited to people with macular disease.

Not Just for the Blind

Does it mean you are blind if you decide to use the services of an organization with the word "blind" in its name? No!

The word "blind" is in the names of many local centers, national nonprofit organizations, and government agencies. Do not be turned off or scared away by that word. Some people have been known to refuse to even contact an agency because the word "blind" is in its title. Could this be a rationalization for not getting help?

Note that many longtime nonprofit organizations have changed their names over the years to indicate that they serve people with varying degrees of low vision. Some agencies now include the words "visually handicapped," "vision loss," or "visually impaired." For example, as mentioned in the My Story on page 142, the center in Minneapolis is now named Vision Loss Resources. It was founded in 1914 as the Minneapolis Society for the Blind and was renamed in 1990 when it merged with another local agency.

Letting Family, Friends, and Strangers Know Your Needs

Your vision loss affects not only you, but your family and friends, too. They may gradually need to help you with various tasks, but let that help be in ways that are appropriate and useful for you. If you are not the instigator of the idea of such help, you can feel a loss of control. Realize that it should be up to you to decide what help you want to accept and when you want to actively seek help in a particular area of your life.

Ideas for Handling Various "Help" Situations

Sometimes family and friends do not know what to do about giving you the help you may—or may not—need. It is up to you to let them know what it right for you. Here are examples of some types of people and how to handle situations with them.

- **Overly protective; offer unsolicited help that you do not need.** You can be politely assertive and say, "It's important that I stay as independent as possible, so please allow me do whatever I can. I'll ask for assistance when I need it, so don't feel you always need to offer help."

- **Oblivious to your situation; ignore the fact that you need assistance in some area—the opposite of being too solicitous.** It is again up to you to let them know what you need. You can say, "I appreciate your thinking I can do everything myself, but I would like your help with (you name it)."

- **Attuned to your needs and desires.** This is the ideal situation, so accept the help with thanks.

- **Persistent in offering help that you could actually use but want to reject because you'd then have to admit that you need it.** This has much less to do with other people than it does with you. Ask yourself, "Am I like some people who let pride or denial get in the way of acting in my own best interests?" If the answer is yes, try not to become huffy, as I did (and came to regret) when I didn't want to accept a ride, as told in the My Story on pages 167–168.

Asking for—or Accepting—Too Much Help

If someone in your life is a very helpful type, it is easy to fall into the trap of automatically accepting or asking for help you do not really need. Doing so will ultimately reduce your independence. In my own case, I need to be more aware so I don't use help from my son that I don't really need. He comes to work every weekday in the home office of our family publishing business. He is patient and kind and, for instance, if I can't find something I've set down somewhere right away, I get frustrated and ask him to find it rather than keep searching for it myself.

Sometimes when I find myself too easily accepting or relying on assistance with some task I could safely accomplish on my own, I remember a gentleman who attended the low vision skills class I took. He had very little vision and his wife drove him to class, but she did not "hang around" during the class to assist him—instead, she went upstairs, did crossword puzzles, and came back in time to join in the lunch we had prepared in class. She reminded him that he was in the class to learn to do things for himself. She was reinforcing his need for independence, and she let him know that she was not going to help him when he could do something for himself. This example serves as a good reminder to be conscious of the type of help we are using and to make sure it is at an appropriate level.

Becoming Proactive in Communicating Your Needs

The ideal is for you to become comfortable in talking to your family and friends about your needs.

- Be open about telling people how you are feeling so they don't have to try to guess whether or not something is wrong.

- If you are having a bad eye day (or, as one woman puts it, "My eyes are crabby today"), you may need to ask for special attention or help in deciding whether or not you should participate in a planned activity.

- Feel free to suggest things you really would like from others, such as offers to take you shopping or to a doctor appointment, or fun things like going out to lunch or the opportunity to show gift ideas that you have found in low vision catalogs.

Recognizing and Reducing Stress

A common reaction to loss—which can include events such as a task taking twice as long to perform as before or a non-event such as beginning to acknowledge that you should stop driving—is stress. The body frequently expresses stress in the forms of headache, stomachache, or trouble sleeping. There will be times when you feel particularly harried or frustrated or sad and want to bury those feelings. Instead, deal with your stress by:

- Talking about it with those around you. If you are alone, call a family member or friend. The important thing is to talk about it.

- Realizing that stress is contagious—if you are feeling stressed, chances are good that everyone around you will also begin to feel stressed. If you are all trying to ignore, deny, or bottle up your feelings, you will end up with a group of inwardly seething, frustrated people.

- Telling people if you are overwhelmed and need help, rather than wondering why they can't see that you are waiting for them to offer it.

- Recognizing that a grief expressed is a grief diminished.

- Taking a break
- Knowing that it's OK to yell or cry
- Helping someone else

The best way to prevent stress from building up is, of course, to prevent it from taking hold in the first place. Here are some ways to ward off stress in your life.

- Know your limits and set realistic goals when you plan your day
- Refuse to hold grudges or feel sorry for yourself
- Get enough sleep
- Exercise regularly
- Meditate or regularly engage in the practices of your belief system
- Laugh often, even if you don't feel like doing so

Talking About Your Vision Loss—It's Up to You

Sometimes when you are out and about, you may run into situations in which it would make sense to mention you have a vision loss. Remember that, in all cases, it is up to you to decide whether or not you want to say anything. Here are some scenarios and ideas on how you could handle them.

At a store, you may need help with reading a price tag, or with signing a charge slip at the checkout station when you can't see the line on which to write your signature. It is a good idea to practice saying a standard line, such as, "Please show me where to sign, as I don't see well (or have vision loss, or have poor vision, or whatever words you prefer), so that you can say it with ease and confidence when necessary.

- At social gatherings, you may want to get into discussions and be more open about your specific condition, such as when the person you are talking to mentions that a relative or friend has vision loss.

- If people become overly inquisitive, remember that you are under no obligation to talk about your vision. You can say, "I prefer not to discuss this," or, even better, "I find it rather boring to discuss my vision loss."

Trying to Identify People

It can be embarrassing when you can't recognize people because you can't make out their faces or see them from across the room. If someone you know comes up to you at a social function and you can't tell who it is by his or her voice, you can explain that you don't see well. Actually, this is a lot better than having to say you have completely forgotten the person's name, which can happen, too, and which is, to my mind, even more embarrassing.

It can be a good idea to ask even people you know well and see often that they make a habit of identifying themselves when they enter the room and telling you when they are leaving.

Develop a Spirit of Gratitude for the Help Your Receive

As we continue to make adjustments in our lives to accommodate our vision loss we can experience many feelings, but gratitude may not readily come to mind. Try to remember to thank the helpers in your life. Let them know you appreciate what they do for you and recognize that your situation makes life difficult for them, too. Sometimes I think I present a triple whammy to those around me—I have vision loss and need help in many areas, I have a hearing loss—and I don't always wear my hearing aids, so I'm often saying, "What? Can you say that again more clearly?" and I have celiac disease and can't eat a normal diet—no wheat, oats, barley, or rye. My family and friends have immense kindness and patience in the ways they must adapt their lives to fit my needs, yet how often do I remember to let them know how grateful I am for their help?

Using Local and Regional Recreational, Transportation, and Medical Resources

Besides your immediate circle of family and friends, there are local resources that can offer you help and a variety of services in the areas of recreation, transportation, and health care. In addition to the special adaptive recreational opportunities described below, assistive services are offered by a wide array of senior centers and community centers, as well as by vision loss agencies that offer a variety of social and recreational activities, which are described later in the chapter.

Adaptive Recreational Opportunities

Audio descriptions of the visual elements of live theater, selected television shows, and some movies are available to enhance your understanding and pleasure of these types of entertainment.

- **Television.** Descriptions by a narrator of visual elements such as actions, settings, scene changes, and body language are provided during natural breaks in the program's dialogue. Check with your local stations or cable companies to see what is available. Also, when buying a new television set, be sure that it can accept audio description.

- **Audio-described performance.** Theater productions of plays that run for long periods of time (as opposed to those that open and close very quickly or that come into town for a day or two) often have performances that include audio descriptions. You wear a headset to hear the narration. Ticket prices are often subsidized for you and a companion. Call your local theater companies to find out if they have these performances.

- **Audio-described movies and videos.** Visit the following Web sites to locate movie theaters that show audio-described films by city, state, and country. You can also call local movie theaters to ask if they show audio-described movies.

    United States: www.dts.com/digitalcinema//dtsaccess/dts_access_locations.php

    Other countries: http://adinternational.org/ADImovies.html#other

A list of audio-described movies with ratings on the ease or difficulty of following the story is offered by the Web site Blindspots: Movie Reviews for Visually Impaired People (www.vashti.net/Blind/table.htm).

Talking Books and Magazines from Your Regional NLS Library

You can borrow recorded books, magazines, and playback equipment from a regional library that is in the network of the Talking Book Program of the National Library Service for the Blind and Physically Handicapped (NLS). The Talking Book Program is discussed more thoroughly in chapter 9, but these key points are worth mentioning again.

- The program is available to U.S. residents and U.S. citizens living abroad whose low vision, blindness, or physical handicap makes it difficult to read a standard printed page. The eligibility requirements of the Talking

Book Program are less stringent than those of the other government agencies listed at the end of this chapter.

- Playback machines for listening to the recordings are provided on free loan.

- The U.S. Postal Service delivers the recordings, which are sent to you from your regional library, and you return them, postage free, to the to the regional library.

- To enroll in the program, you can start the process by calling 1-888-657-7323 and following the prompts to be connected to the appropriate library. You can also find your library and fill out a request form on the NLS Web site (www.loc.gov/nls.index.html).

- Your local vision loss agency can help you with your application by leading you through the process and helping you fill out the forms.

Transportation Services

Information on transportation services for the disabled is mentioned at the end of chapter 10. Under the provisions of the Americans with Disabilities Act (ADA) of 1990, most communities provide special transportation services for people with disabilities, including those with vision loss. To find transportation services in your area, contact your local Area Agency on Aging by calling 1-800-677-1116. Note, too, that many telephone directories have sections in the front of the books with the names and addresses of various service organizations—some phone books may include information on transportation services for people with special needs.

Medical Specialists

Put together a medical team that will cover all aspects of your health care, starting with your primary care physician, who will take care of your basic health needs and refer you to specialists for specific conditions. Below is a list of some of the specialists who may become part of your personal health care team.

- **Retinologist.** Your retinologist is an essential member of your team. It is important to keep your routine appointments, and it is crucial that you see your retinologist whenever you notice a change in your vision because there may be a benefit from an early treatment.

- **Ophthalmologist.** You will see your ophthalmologist once a year for a general eye checkup and to explore the possibility of improving your vision with a new eyeglass prescription.

- **Ophthalmic plastic surgeon.** If you wish to explore the possibility of surgery to correct drooping eyelids that are blocking your field of vision, this is the specialist you should consult. First, get the opinions of your ophthalmologist and retinologist, and get a referral if you want to pursue the idea.

- **Occupational therapist.** To help maximize your independence in your daily activities, an occupational therapist can provide evaluation and training services to help you live with your vision loss. See the entry for the American Occupational Therapy Association in the organization list on pages 193–194 for more information.

- **Physical therapist.** Balance and physical fitness are especially important for people with vision loss, and a physical therapist can develop an exercise program to fit your particular needs.

- **Podiatrist.** A large number of balance problems originate in the feet, and a podiatrist may suggest you get orthotic aids to put in your shoes for extra support. A podiatrist can also provide toenail care and remove painful corns and calluses that may be making it difficult to walk.

- **Your own specialists.** Depending on your own health conditions, you may see specialists in various fields, such as an endocrinologist if you have diabetes.

Deciding to Seek Help from Local Vision Loss Organizations

You may be lucky enough to live in a community that has a vision loss agency—these organizations can offer you a wealth of services. Realize that it can be scary to even start thinking about looking for help outside your own circle. You may feel that, by acknowledging your need for more help than friends and family can give, you are surrendering your independence. Just the opposite is true, as you will learn new ways to remain independent and maximize control over your life. Perhaps you feel uncomfortable about the prospect of sharing your story with strangers or about taking a class for the first time in years. But making that first call is a very positive step, because it shows that you are accepting your condition to the point that you are ready to open the doors to whole new ways of living.

What Will Happen When I Call?

The first step when you call will be to set up an appointment for an intake interview. At this interview basic identification information will be gathered, and you may be asked about the history of your disease. In some cases, a staff person will also do a simple functional vision evaluation to get an idea of the equipment and services that might be helpful for you.

What Services Will I Be Offered?

You will probably meet with a counselor, who will tell you about the various services that are offered at the center. Examples, from the huge variety of activities that may be offered, are listed below, but understand that not all organizations will offer all of these services.

- **Computer training**

  Accessibility software for magnifying what is on the screen and for reading aloud what is on the screen.

  Communicating by e-mail

  Keyboard typing skills

- **Cooking**

  Adaptive cooking and kitchen safety techniques

  Recipes in large type

  Special kitchen aids

- **Daily living skills**

  Doing household chores

  Handling money

  Managing finances

  Marking and identifying clothing and other items

  Organizing household items and furniture

- **Fitness and health**

  Guidance in designing a personalized fitness program

  Healthy-eating support groups

  Instruction on using fitness equipment

  Yoga and workout classes

  Walking groups

- **Filling out forms**

  Assistance with filling out forms such as applications for Talking Books or mobility services

  Help with filling out income tax returns

- **In-home evaluation**

  Development of a plan of service

  Identification of needs for magnifiers, lighting, etc.

  Information on other community resources

- **Leisure and recreation**

  Craft classes and groups in such areas as basket weaving, woodworking, soap making, and jewelry making

  Needlework classes and groups in such areas as knitting, crocheting, and quilting

  Bingo, cribbage, and board games

  Book clubs that use books on tape

  Card games such as hearts, bridge, and poker

  Journal and creative writing classes and groups

  Lunch and supper club outings

  Movie showings with audio descriptions

  Trips to museums and plays

- **Library**

  Audio books

Audio-described videos and DVDs

Large print periodicals and books

- **Support groups**

  Support and socialization with peers who understand your challenges, meeting in groups moderated by a staff person or a trained volunteer facilitator

- **Volunteers and volunteering**

  Help with shopping, reading, and leisure skills

  One-on-one peer counseling with trained, visually impaired volunteers

  Opportunities to become a volunteer yourself!

- **Miscellaneous**

  Free Bible on tape

  Free directory assistance for your telephone

  Large print or amplified phones, if you also have hearing loss

  Mobility transportation services

  Talking Books, radio, and newspaper reading services

What Services Are Offered to the Community?

Many low vision agencies offer community education by providing speakers for people living in various types of residences, such as assisted living or long-term care faculties, and to members of organizations such as senior centers. If you would like to arrange for a speaker for your group, contact your local agency. Many low vision agencies also have speakers who provide information on vision loss to other professionals.

MY STORY

Why Did It Take Me So Long?

I keep notes of every visit with my retinologist, and every now and then I remembered making a note about a counselor at Vision Loss Resources, a local vision rehabilitation agency, whom the doctor had mentioned on more than one visit. That first time the counselor was mentioned I remember having asked if there were any support groups, so the referral was in response to my question. I just kept the idea of calling the counselor pretty well buried in the back of my mind until my retinologist brought it up again during other visits. Still, I did nothing.

When I finally made the call to the counselor, I checked my notes and found that it had been four years since the doctor first told me about her. By then it had been eight years since my initial diagnosis. The benefits of meeting with the counselor have been enormous. Perhaps the most important benefit is that, by taking that first step, I finally had become ready to go after help on my own.

At that first meeting I kept hearing peals of laughter from the next room, and I was invited to join the group of men and women who were having a wonderful time eating the lunch that the cooking instructor had prepared in a demonstration. The people in this group had very severe vision loss. I was seated next to two women who were members of the organization's advocacy group and who were involved in community education. They go out to various facilities and tell groups about the services offered by the center. The women also had received training to become para-professional aides to assist the staff members who moderate support groups. These inspiring women showed me how much someone with severe macular disease could contribute, even when living with only peripheral vision.

Enrolling as a client at the center has changed my life. My resolve to keep a positive outlook has been affirmed and bolstered by meetings with my counselor, and other staff members have guided me in various ways. I have met inspiring people with vision loss in classes and at various functions at the center. In a weekly life skills class I learned many new ways to live my life, including special cooking techniques, how-to ideas for that all-important organization I need in my life, and an upbeat approach to dealing with the frustrations of living with vision loss.

Why did I wait so long to take the first step in seeking help? My counselor tells me that it was because I was not ready earlier. She said that people come at all stages of their disease, and that there is not a single "right" time for everyone—the right time is when one is ready. Sometimes I wish I had been ready earlier, but I think a streak of stubbornness got in my way. When others in my class who were at later stages of vision loss had difficulty reading the recipes printed in giant-size type, I kept thinking, "If only they had come sooner, they could have been using these practical ideas for years." Then I remembered that the same wisdom applies to me.

National Nonprofit Organizations— Programs and Services

There are an estimated 1,400 agencies across the United States devoted to helping individuals and their families adapt to living with vision loss. Some of the nonprofit agencies that provide important advocacy, education, and research functions, as well as especially useful services to people with macular disease, are described below. The specific services fall into two categories:

- Locators that provide assistance in finding specific services in your community, such as chapters of national organizations, state services, talking radio stations, and many others.

- Publications that feature news of the latest research developments and that list centers for computer training.

Browse the list to find an organization that appeals to your interests, then contact the service to find out what it can do for you.

American Foundation for the Blind (AFB)

11 Penn Plaza, Suite 300, New York, NY 10001
Phone: 800-232-5463
E-mail: afbinfo@afb.net
Web site: www.afb.org
Find a service near you: www.afb.org/seniorsitedir.asp

The AFB's mission is to broaden access to technology, elevate the quality of information and tools for the professionals who serve people with vision loss, promote independent and healthy living for people with vision loss by providing them and their families relevant and timely resources, and maintain a strong presence in Washington, DC, to ensure that the rights and interests of people with vision loss are represented in our nation's public policies.

The AFB Web site has an online directory of more than 1,500 organizations in the United States and Canada that provide services such as computer training, counseling, support groups, and classes in independent living skills. You can search by all or specific types of service after selecting your state or province. The AFB Web site also features candid reviews of new adaptive technology products—you can read these reviews by going to www.afb.org/Section.asp?SectionID=4&TopicID=31 and clicking on "AFB Product Evaluations."

American Macular Degeneration Foundation (AMDF)

PO Box 515, Northampton, MA 01061
Phone: 888-622-8527
E-mail: amdf@macular.org
Web site: www.macular.org
Find a state agency: www.macular.org/stagency/index.html
Publication: The newsletter *SPOTLIGHT* provides scientific information about macular degeneration.

The American Macular Degeneration Foundation works for the prevention, treatment, and cure of macular degeneration by raising funds, educating the public, and supporting scientific research. Services include vocational rehabilitation and job placement services, financial assistance or referrals to other agencies or organizations that provide similar services in the community, orientation and mobility training, and transportation services.

The AMDF's Web site lists the government agency in each state that provides services to the blind and visually impaired.

American Occupational Therapy Association, Inc. (AOTA)

4720 Montgomery Lane, PO Box 31220
Bethesda, MD 20824
Phone: 301-652-2682

Web site: www.aota.org
Find a driving evaluator: www.aota.org/driver_search/index.aspx

The AOTA is an official association of professional occupational therapists throughout the United States. If there is no specialized vision loss agency in your area, consider securing the services of an occupational therapist—he or she can help you with many of the things you would learn at a specialized agency, including cooking, marking items for easy identification, developing senses besides sight, and using assistive devices. These services are provided in your home, and suggestions could be made about your lighting and furniture arrangements. Through the AOTA Web site, you can even find an occupational therapist that can perform a driving evaluation if you or your family have concerns about your current ability. Any occupational therapist will be able to help you with your tasks of everyday living, and you may find a therapist in your community who has had training in the AOTA specialty of assisting older adults with low vision.

Community Services for the Blind and Partially Sighted (CSBPS)

9709 Third Avenue NE, #100, Seattle, WA 98115
Phone: 800-458-4888
E-mail: csbps@csbps.com
Web site: http://csbps.com

Publication: *PRISM*, a large print newsletter published quarterly, features news and information for blind and visually impaired people and their families, senior organizations, health care professionals, financial contributors, and others. It is available free of charge online, on audiocassette, and in braille.

Founded in 1965 as a private, nonprofit agency, CSBPS provides rehabilitation services to people with low vision in three counties in the state of Washington. It sells products nationwide through its Sight Connection store. Visit the CSBPS Web site for a link to the store's current catalog.

Foundation Fighting Blindness (FFB)

11435 Cronhill Drive, Owings Mills, MD 21117
Phone: 800-683-5555
E-mail: info@FightBlindness.org
Web site: www.blindness.org
Find a local chapter: www.blindness.org/content.asp?id=5

The mission of the FFB is to drive research that will lead to the prevention, treatment, and cure of retinal disease. FFP has funded thousands of research studies at hundreds of prominent institutions worldwide, including leading-edge research in promising areas such as genetics, gene therapy, retinal cell transplantation, artificial retinal implants, and pharmaceutical and nutritional therapies. In addition, the FFB provides information and outreach programs for patients, families, and professionals. More than 50 volunteer-led groups across the United States raise funds, increase public awareness, and provide support to each other and their communities. The FFB was named one of *Worth* magazine's "100 Best Charities."

The FFB Web site features special pages on retinitis pigmentosa, macular degeneration, Usher syndrome, and a large spectrum of other retinal degenerative diseases. Each of these pages provides information on the particular disease, as well as information on current research activities.

International Association of Audio Information Services (IAAIS)

Phone: 800-280-5325
Web site: http://iaais.org/aboutiaais.html
Find a radio station: http://iaais.org/locateservice.html

The IAAIS is a volunteer-driven organization of services that turn text into speech for those who are unable to read or hold printed material. Many U.S. members of IAAIS are associated with public radio stations, colleges and universities, and libraries.

The organization works actively to promote and protect access to all forms of information available to the general public. As part of its services, the IAAIS maintains a directory of radio stations that provide immediate, verbatim audio access to newspapers, magazines, consumer information, and other materials. Topic-based and public affairs programs are also available on many stations, as are some books and story-based programs. In addition, some IAAIS members' services include a variety of related programs, such as personal reader programs; audio-description services of live theater, museum exhibits, nature trails, parades, and other visual venues; audio transcription; taping services; and other audio-based community services.

Lions Clubs International

300 W 22nd Street, Oak Brook, IL 60523
Phone: 630-571-5466, x383 (Foundation Division)
E-mail: lcif@lionsclubs.org
Web site: www.lionsclubs.org/EN/index.shtml
Find a local club: www.lionsclubs.org/EN/content/about_index.shtml#

The Foundation Division of the Lions Clubs administers the Sight Conservation and Work with the Blind program. It has several projects that aid the visually impaired, including several rehabilitation centers in the United States.

Local clubs may sponsor programs for the visually impaired and may donate aids such as talking clocks and, sometimes, computers to people who are visually impaired. Some clubs provide large print books to libraries.

Macular Degeneration Partnership

8733 Beverly Boulevard, #201, Los Angeles, CA 90048
Phone: 888-430-9898
Web site: www.amd.org
Publication: *AMD News Update*, an e-mail newsletter, features excellent information regarding current research on both the dry and wet forms of macular degeneration

The Macular Degeneration Partnership is an outreach program of the nonprofit Discovery Eye Foundation. Its mission is to provide comprehensive, easily understood, and up-to-the-minute information about macular degeneration to the public through the Internet, telephone, public events, and printed materials. The organization's goal is to support research and to coordinate advocacy efforts.

The Macular Disease Society (United Kingdom)

PO Box 1870, Andover, SP10 9AD, ENGLAND
Phone: 01264 350551
E-mail: info@maculardisease.org
Web site: http://maculardiseaseorg.site.securepod.com/default.asp
Publication: The magazine *Side View*, which is published quarterly, is written by members for members and is available in large print or on audiocassette. Its content is wide ranging and includes articles on macular disease, low vision aids, the latest developments in macular

disease research, and news from the society's wide group of U.K. members.

This British organization is a self-help society for those diagnosed with any of the eye conditions that fall under the classification of macular disease. The society is dedicated to providing information and practical support so that those with the condition may make the most of their remaining vision.

National Association for Visually Handicapped (NAVH)

22 West 21st Street, 6th Floor, New York, NY 10010
Phone: 212-255-2804
E-mail: navh@navh.org
Web site: www.navh.org
Publication: *NAVH Update* is a free newsletter, published quarterly, that covers the latest information on eye disease, assistive aids and lighting, and nutrition. It is available via mail and e-mail; visit the NAVH Web site to request a subscription.

The NAVH provides public education on limited vision through outreach programs and professional information at conferences. Its Large Print Loan Library has one of the nation's largest collections of large print books for loan. The service is free to members, and the books are mailed anywhere in the United States. Most of the books in this library carry the prestigious NAVH Seal of Approval and are donated by publishers who use the large print standards that NAVH pioneered. A catalog of titles is available free to members and for a $6 donation by non-members.

Prevent Blindness America

211 West Wacker Drive, Suite 1700, Chicago, Illinois 60606
Phone: 1-800-331-2020
E-mail: info@preventblindness.org
Web site: www.preventblindness.org
Find an affiliate: www.preventblindness.org/about/affiliates.html

Founded in 1908, Prevent Blindness America is a volunteer eye health and safety organization whose sole mission is the prevention of blindness and the preservation of sight. The organization offers education programs, screenings for vision problems in adults at locations such as senior centers and for vision problems in children in schools, training and certification for people around the country to conduct screenings, and various community and patient service programs, including an e-mail newsletter. Prevent Blindness America advocates at the local, state, and national levels to promote sound public policy and adequate funding for initiatives that prevent blindness and save sight. Its annual "Eyes on Capitol Hill" event provides vision advocates an opportunity to meet with congressional leaders and policymakers.

The organization's Web site features pages on diabetic retinopathy and macular degeneration, a list of affiliate groups in several states, and other information for people with vision loss.

SeniorNet

900 Lafayette Street, Suite 604, Santa Clara, CA 95050
Phone: 408-615-0699
Web site: www.seniornet.org
Find a Learning Center: www.seniornet.org/jsnet/ index.php?option=com_content&task=view&id=64&Item id=94

SeniorNet provides older adults education and access to computer technologies to enhance their lives and enable them to share their knowledge and wisdom. The organization supports about 200 Learning Centers throughout the United States and in other countries. These centers offer courses on introductions to computers, word processing, the Internet, and e-mail, plus advanced courses on specialized topics. The centers are housed in a variety of locations such as senior centers, community centers, public libraries, schools and colleges, and clinics and hospitals. SeniorNet also offers easy-to-understand online lessons in using a computer, including utilizing accessibility options. In addition, the organization offers discounts on computer-related and other products and services.

SeniorNet publishes newsletters and a variety of other instructional materials. It collaborates in research on older adults and technology, and it holds regional conferences for volunteers.

Government Agencies— Programs, Services, and Eligibility

The Assistive Technology Act, enacted by Congress in 1998, is commonly known as the "Tech Act." Today, funding authorized by the Tech Act supports three general types of programs, which vary from state to state: grant programs, protection and advocacy services, and alternative financing programs for purchasing assistive technology. The Tech Act provides services to those who live with virtually any type of disability for these people's full lifespans.

Some government agencies have special programs for people who are eligible for services if they meet their strict definition of "blind." If you meet one of the following criteria, you may qualify for these programs.

- Even with glasses or contact lenses, you cannot see better than 20/200 in your better eye
- Your field of vision is 20 degrees or less

Although people with macular disease may never reach this stage of vision loss, information on some of the major programs is included here nevertheless. It is possible that there could be some flexibility in applying the criteria.

Department of Veterans Affairs, Blind Rehabilitation Service

Director, Blind Rehabilitation Service
Department of Veterans Affairs Central Office
810 Vermont Avenue NW, Washington, DC 20420
Phone: 202-273-9163
Web site: www.va.gov
Find a facility: www1.va.gov/directory/guide/home.asp?isFlash=1

If you are a veteran and meet the criteria of the Blind Rehabilitation Service, you are eligible to receive services through this organization. The Visual Impairment Service Team (VIST) coordinator serves as the initial contact person for getting help for your vision loss and to ensure that veterans with vision impairments receive appropriate benefits and services. VIST coordinators are located at local VA medical centers across the country. To find the facility nearest you, visit the organization's Web site or contact your county veteran's service officer.

Training programs are available in the following areas.

- Visual skills devices, including special electronic viewing devices that supplement optical low vision devices
- Communication devices, including electronic reading machines, computers, and other similar specialized devices

- Electronic orientation and mobility devices that supplement the usual protective travel devices such as the long cane

Internal Revenue Service

Phone: 800-829-1040
Web site: www.irs.gov/publications/p554/ch04.html#d0e2715

If you meet the IRS's criteria for eligibility, you can receive an income tax reduction for blindness that is equal to the deduction for being over 65 years old. To claim the deduction for "partly blind," you must have a statement, certified by your eye doctor or registered optometrist, that declares one of the following:

- Even with glasses or contact lenses, you cannot see better than 20/200 in your better eye, or;

- Your field of vision is 20 degrees or less

For many older and visually impaired taxpayers, the "over 65" and "blind" deductions result in more of a tax break than they would get if they itemized deductions, including expenses incurred as a result of vision impairment. And they definitely require a lot less work on the tax form than itemizing.

Centers for Medicare and Medicaid Services

7500 Security Boulevard, Baltimore, MD 21244
Phone: 800-633-4227
Web site: www.cms.hhs.gov

Services covered by Medicare depend on the specific plan you have and whether or not you are also covered by Medicaid. Coverage varies from plan to plan, but services may include doctor visits, prescription drug coverage, coverage of costs incurred with eye injections, surgery for drooping eyelids or eyebrows, and mobility training. Check with your provider for information on the vision-related services that are covered in your plan.

National Eye Institute (NEI), Information Office, National Institutes of Health

31 Center Drive MSC 2510, Bethesda, MD 20892
Phone: 301-496-5248
E-mail: 2020@nei.nih.gov
Web site: www.nei.nih.gov

The NEI was founded by Congress in 1968. It conducts research and education programs and provides information on eye diseases. The National Eye Institute's Office of Communication, Health Education, and Public Liaison responds directly to requests for information on eye diseases and vision research.

State Commission of the Blind

Find services near you: www.macular.org/stagency/index.html

The name of this organization varies by state—it is also known as State Services for the Blind and Visually Handicapped, Division of Rehabilitation Services; Blind Services, Department of Human Services; Aid to the Aged, Blind or Disabled; and other names. Each state provides services to the visually handicapped, but the governmental organizations themselves and the services they provide vary from state to state.

Services that may be provided include:

- Vocational rehabilitation and job placement services
- Financial assistance or referrals to other agencies and organizations that provide similar services in the community
- Orientation and mobility training and transportation
- Communication center that has a special library and transcription service, providing reading material in alternate formats to citizens who have difficulty reading normal print
- Provision of playback machines for the Talking Book Program

Appendix A

Suppliers of Low Vision Products

ALMOST ALL of the products mentioned in this book are available at one or more of the three low vision stores listed below. There may also be local stores in your community where you can see and buy some of the products. Information on where to purchase products not available from the three stores is provided here.

Low Vision Stores

independent living aids, inc.
PO Box 9022, Hicksville, NY 11802
Phone: 800-537-2118
Web site: www.independentliving.com

LS&S

1808-G Janke Drive, Northbrook, IL 60062

Phone: 800-468-4789

Web site: www.lssproducts.com

Maxi-Aids, Inc.

42 Executive Boulevard, Farmingdale, NY 11735

Phone: 800-522-6294

Web site: www.maxiaids.com

Hard-to-Find Products Mentioned in This Book

The following specific brands and products can be hard to find, so purchasing information is given below. Often the easiest way to get these items is through a Web site that sells a wide variety of products, such as Amazon.com (www.amazon.com). If you are not a computer user, ask a relative or friend to order for you.

Flashlite Friend™

Nite Ize, Inc.

5660 Central Avenue, Boulder, CO 80301

Phone: 800-678-6483

Web site: www.niteize.com/productdetail.php?category_id=28&product_id=62

Giraffe Lamp
Goodwin Manufacturing, Inc.
PO Box 5981, High Point, NC 27262
Phone: 800-282-5267
Web site: www.giraffelamps.com/low.htm

Jitterbug® cell phone
Jitterbug by GreatCall, Inc.
Phone: 800-918-8543
Web site: www.jitterbug.com

'Ove' Glove®
This is available at various cooking and housewares stores, as well as at the "As Seen On TV" Web site (www. asseenontv.com/prod-pages/ove_glove.html).

Stainless steel measuring cups and spoons
These are available at various cooking and housewares stores, as well as at Amazon.com (search for "metal measuring cups").

Appendix B

Manufacturers and Distributors of Assistive Technology Products

THE PRODUCTS described in chapter 9 are generally available from at least one of the three low vision stores listed in Appendix A. This Appendix B contains a list of representative manufacturers and U.S. distributors of these products as of this writing. If you are outside the United States, visit the companies' Web sites to obtain phone numbers, e-mail addresses, and other contact information that pertains to your country.

Assistive technology is developing at such a rapid pace, with a steady stream of new products coming to market, that any list of specific products available is likely to become outdated very quickly. Use the contact information below to help you find the latest devices and software that are currently on the market from these companies. (Note that some manufacturers are listed more than once because they make products in more than one category.) You can also consult the AFB's (American Foundation for the Blind) Web site for excellent, up-to-date lists of products and manufacturers. The AFB's Web site also features reviews of new products—you can find them online by going to www.afb.org/Section.asp?SectionID=4&TopicID=31 and clicking on "AFB Product Evaluations."

Scanner Readers, Desktop

Guerilla Technologies
5029 SE Horseshoe Point Road, Stuart, FL 34997
Phone: 772-283-0500
Web site: www.guerillatechnologies.com

Scanner Readers, Portable

Enhanced Vision
Phone: 888-811-3161
E-mail: evinfo@enhancedvision.com
Web site: www.enhancedvision.com

K-NFB Reading Technology, Inc.
PO Box 620128, Newton Lower Falls, MA 02462
Phone: 877-547-1500
Web site: www.knfbreader.com

Kurzweil Educational Systems, Inc.
100 Crosby Drive, Bedford, MA 01730
Phone: 800-894-5374
E-mail: info@kurzweiledu.com
Web site: www.kurzweiledu.com

Scanner Readers/Magnifiers, Portable Multifunction

Guerilla Technologies
5029 SE Horseshoe Point Road, Stuart, FL 34997
Phone: 772-283-0500
Web site: www.guerillatechnologies.com

Software, Internet-Access (No Typing Required)

Serotek Corporation
1128 Harmon Place, Suite 310, Minneapolis, MN 55403
Phone: 866-202-0520
E-mail: info@serotek.com
Web site: www.serotek.com

Software, Magnification/Screen Reading (Typing Required)

Ai Squared
This company produces both screen magnification and screen reading software.
PO Box 669, Manchester Center, VT 05255
Phone: 800-859-0270
E-mail: sales@aisquared.com
Web site: www.aisquared.com

Dolphin Computer Access, Ltd.
(Headquarters: United Kingdom)
This company produces both screen magnification and screen reading software.
Phone: 866-797-5921
E-mail: info@dolphinusa.com
Web site: www.yourdolphin.com

Freedom Scientific
This company produces both screen magnification and screen reading software.
11800 31st Court North, St. Petersburg, FL 33716
Phone: 800-202-0520
E-mail: info@freedomscientific.com
Web site: www.freedomscientific.com

Software, Speech Recognition

Mac Speech, Inc.
50A Northwestern Drive, Suite 109, Salem, NH 03079
Phone: 603-350-0903
Web site: www.macspeech.com

Nuance
1 Wayside Road, Burlington, MA 01803
Phone: 781-565-5000
Web site: www.nuance.com

Video Magnifiers (CCTVs)

Ash Technologies, Ltd.
(Headquarters: Ireland)
U.S. distributor: Freedom Vision
Phone: 800-961-1334
E-mail: info@freedomvision.net
Web site: www.freedomvision.net

Human Ware
(Headquarters: Australia)
Phone: 800-722-3393
E-mail: us.info@humanware.com
Web site: www.humanware.com/en-usa/home

Low Vision International
(Headquarters: Sweden)
Find contact information for the distributor nearest you by visiting the company's Web site.
Web site: www.lvi.se/sprak/eng/index.htm

Optelec
(Headquarters: Netherlands)
Phone: 800-828-1056
Web site: www.optelec.com

Video Magnifiers, Handheld, That Plug into TVs and Computers (CCTVs)

Bierley
(Headquarters: United Kingdom)
Phone: 800-985-0535
E-mail: info@bierley.com
Web site: www.bierley.com

Enhanced Vision
Phone: 888-811-3161
E-mail: evinfo@enhancedvision.com
Web site: www.enhancedvision.com

Index